MW00634653

MEDITERRANEAN
PRESSURE COOKING

MEDITERRANEAN
PRESSURE COOKING

Vibrant Mediterranean Diet Recipes
for Any Electric Pressure Cooker

ABBIE GELLMAN, MS, RD, CDN

Photography by Andrew Purcell

ROCKRIDGE
PRESS

Copyright © 2020 by Rockridge Press, Emeryville, California

No part of this publication may be reproduced, stored in a retrieval system, or transmitted in any form or by any means, electronic, mechanical, photocopying, recording, scanning, or otherwise, except as permitted under Sections 107 or 108 of the 1976 United States Copyright Act, without the prior written permission of the Publisher. Requests to the Publisher for permission should be addressed to the Permissions Department, Rockridge Press, 6005 Shellmound Street, Suite 175, Emeryville, CA 94608.

Limit of Liability/Disclaimer of Warranty: The Publisher and the author make no representations or warranties with respect to the accuracy or completeness of the contents of this work and specifically disclaim all warranties, including without limitation warranties of fitness for a particular purpose. No warranty may be created or extended by sales or promotional materials. The advice and strategies contained herein may not be suitable for every situation. This work is sold with the understanding that the Publisher is not engaged in rendering medical, legal, or other professional advice or services. If professional assistance is required, the services of a competent professional person should be sought. Neither the Publisher nor the author shall be liable for damages arising herefrom. The fact that an individual, organization, or website is referred to in this work as a citation and/or potential source of further information does not mean that the author or the Publisher endorses the information the individual, organization, or website may provide or recommendations they/it may make. Further, readers should be aware that websites listed in this work may have changed or disappeared between when this work was written and when it is read.

For general information on our other products and services or to obtain technical support, please contact our Customer Care Department within the United States at (866) 744-2665, or outside the United States at (510) 253-0500.

Rockridge Press publishes its books in a variety of electronic and print formats. Some content that appears in print may not be available in electronic books, and vice versa.

TRADEMARKS: Rockridge Press and the Rockridge Press logo are trademarks or registered trademarks of Callisto Media Inc. and/or its affiliates, in the United States and other countries, and may not be used without written permission. All other trademarks are the property of their respective owners. Rockridge Press is not associated with any product or vendor mentioned in this book.

Interior and Cover Designer: Regina Stadnik
Art Producer: Hannah Dickerson
Editor: Rachelle Cihonski

Photography © 2020 Andrew Purcell, food styling by Carrie Purcell.
All illustrations used under license from Shutterstock.com

ISBN: Print 978-1-64739-836-1 | eBook 978-1-64739-533-9
R0

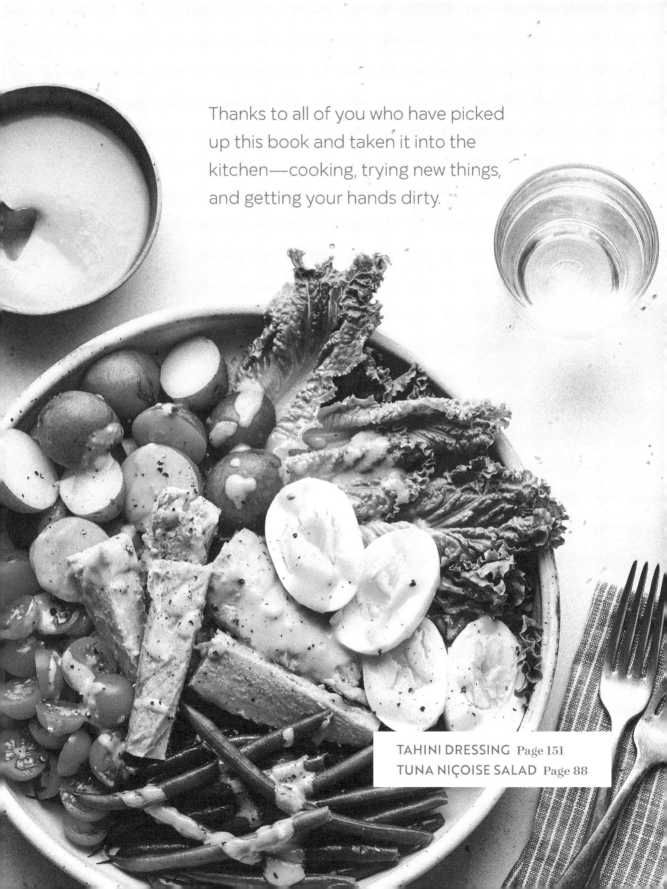

Thanks to all of you who have picked up this book and taken it into the kitchen—cooking, trying new things, and getting your hands dirty.

TAHINI DRESSING Page 151
TUNA NIÇOISE SALAD Page 88

CONTENTS

MOROCCAN TAGINE WITH BUTTERNUT
  SQUASH AND CHICKPEAS Page 68
POACHED PEARS WITH CARDAMOM Page 132
GREEN BEANS WITH CHRAIMEH SAUCE Page 40

INTRODUCTION

I love food. As a chef and registered dietitian, I have a passion for making food that is both healthy and delicious. It is this tenet—along with the idea that food should bring joy and help foster community—that I keep in mind when I create recipes and cook to feed and nourish myself and others.

The Mediterranean diet is a relatively simple style of eating and cooking that I have followed for years. It focuses on using fresh, whole foods, such as fruits, vegetables, beans, and lean protein, and brings an abundance of flavor from a variety of herbs and spices. It is straightforward recipes with these ingredients that empower the readers and viewers of my videos and website, ChefAbbieGellman.com.

I also love my electric pressure cooker and have found it to be an invaluable appliance, especially when I am following a Mediterranean diet. The overall convenience and adaptability have made it a workhorse in many a modern kitchen. My favorite part is that the electric pressure cooker makes healthy cooking easy, tasty, and—best of all—efficient!

As you make your way through this book, you can expect to find a few things. First, there are guidelines and general information regarding the Mediterranean diet and lifestyle. This book will also include information about the electric pressure cooker, including how to use it and other appliance specifics, safety and troubleshooting tips, and helpful tools and accessories.

Finally, there will be dozens of easy, delicious, and healthy Mediterranean diet recipes made with accessible ingredients that can be found at your local grocery store or, in some cases, ordered online. These recipes will focus on whole foods, and many can be enjoyed even if you have dietary restrictions, such as dairy-free or gluten-free. Each recipe will include tips that provide helpful information, swap ideas, shortcuts, or freezing tips, and nutritional information.

Thanks for joining me in the Mediterranean kitchen with your electric pressure cooker. I hope you love these recipes and the Mediterranean diet as much as I do and that this book becomes an integral part of your kitchen and cooking experience. Happy pressure cooking!

CHAPTER ONE

PRESSURE COOKING THROUGH THE MEDITERRANEAN

SPAGHETTI SQUASH WITH CHERRY
TOMATOES, BASIL, AND FETA Page 72

Eating the Mediterranean Way

The Mediterranean diet, ranked as the number one best diet overall and the number one best plant-based diet by *U.S. News & World Report* in 2019 and 2020, is relatively simple in nature. It places an emphasis on eating a variety of whole foods, such as vegetables, whole grains, nuts, and lean protein, and is primarily plant-based, which means that there is a larger emphasis placed on the consumption of plant-based foods than animal-based foods.

Although some diets are extremely rigid, the Mediterranean diet instead provides simple guidelines for improving your eating habits without leaving you feeling deprived or restricted. It is more of a lifestyle and way of thinking that extends beyond just food. On a Mediterranean diet, we can achieve health and wellness with a long-term, holistic view of eating, moving, and living that helps prevent the onset of chronic disease and promote longevity.

So, what exactly does that mean? Here are five main tenets of the Mediterranean diet and lifestyle.

1. **Health Without Sacrifice**
    The Mediterranean diet focuses on nourishing, nutritious ingredients without sacrificing flavor. There are no rules about certain foods being "off limits" or "forbidden." Instead, the emphasis is on moderation.

2. **Quality Over Quantity**
    The Mediterranean diet is a plant-based approach to eating centered on an abundance of fresh whole foods, ranging from fruits and vegetables to nuts and legumes and lean animal proteins like dairy and seafood. It prioritizes choosing quality over quantity, so in general, the portion sizes may be smaller than the standard American or Western diet, but the quality of the food will shine through and leave you satisfied.

3. **Cultivating Community**
    The pleasures of cooking and enjoying a meal among family and friends go hand in hand. The Mediterranean diet and lifestyle is not only about food but also about community, sharing meals with others, and spending time together. Part of cultivating community also includes slowing down to truly enjoy meals and appreciating indulgences like red wine in moderation.

4. **Preserving Culture and Tradition**
The Mediterranean diet is about not only ingredients and recipes but also people, their lives, and where they live. It is steeped in tradition, highlighting flavors and foods that have been passed down through generations as a way of preserving memories and culture.

5. **Staying Active**
Staying physically active and moving is crucial for optimal health and wellness and is a staple of the Mediterranean lifestyle. All physical movement counts, from doing yoga to taking a walk or going for a leisurely swim. Exercise and activity do not have to be competitive or strenuous; the point is to move your body every day.

Paradise Meets the Pressure Cooker

The modern electric pressure cooker is a great way to get you started on the Mediterranean diet. Here are my top reasons why this dynamic duo can give you a push in the right direction.

Healthy meals with less effort: Many people do not want to spend hours prepping and cooking meals on a regular basis. Enter the electric pressure cooker. The majority of recipes in this book are made fully in the electric pressure cooker, so once all the ingredients are sealed in the pot, you simply set it and walk away. Many conventional cooking methods require constant supervision or more hands-on cooking time in addition to the up-front prep time. The electric pressure cooker allows you to skip that and still have delicious, healthy meals regularly.

Redefines "fast food": Many stews, braises, and other dishes that typically take a long time to cook can be made quickly in the electric pressure cooker. Those of us who always feel like we're short on time or simply don't want to spend hours in the kitchen can make a wide variety of healthy, delicious homemade meals without limitations.

More flavorful meals: Pressure cooking creates a closed environment so flavor molecules cannot escape the way they might in a conventional cooking method. A reduced amount of added liquid in an electric pressure cooker recipe is also a means to concentrate flavor. In the case of animal proteins, such as whole chickens or cuts of meat, the natural juices stay put, resulting in juicy, flavorful meat and poultry.

Saves you money: In many instances, electric pressure cookers take less time to cook food compared to other conventional methods and do not use a stovetop or oven. Pressure cookers use 50 to 75 percent less energy, according to the American Council for an Energy-Efficient Economy. Shortened cooking times and less energy use translate to lower energy bills and more money in your pocket. In addition, there are many foods, such as dried beans and legumes, that are cheaper than their canned counterparts and are used frequently in the Mediterranean diet.

How Electric Pressure Cooking Works

An electric pressure cooker can be a helpful addition to the modern kitchen and the Mediterranean lifestyle if you know how to use it. Pressure cookers function based on one overarching principle: that the temperature of boiling liquid is higher in an enclosed, tightly sealed environment. As a result, the time it takes to boil, braise, or steam is greatly reduced.

Once the pressure cooker lid is sealed, locked in place, and turned on, steam develops and cannot escape. These trapped water molecules increase the pressure inside the electric pressure cooker by an average of 12 to 15 pounds per square inch (psi), or 12 to 15 pounds above normal sea level pressure, which raises the boiling point of water from 212°F to between 244°F and 250°F. Depending on the model, electric pressure cookers may have different setting options. A "low" setting of about 5 to 10 psi, or 227°F to 240°F, may be helpful for more delicate foods like puddings or coddled eggs.

Pressure cooking allows you to make healthy, flavorful dishes using whole foods in less time, with minimal cleanup, and often with less oil or added fat. And here's a bonus: Food cooked in the pressure cooker retains more nutrients than boiled food since there's less liquid for vitamins and minerals to leech out into!

THE MEDITERRANEAN REGION

The Mediterranean region, encompassing more than 20 countries, is diverse from both a cultural and culinary point of view. There's no singular diet eaten by all the countries that border the Mediterranean Sea. Instead of specific dishes, the Mediterranean diet focuses on the abundance of healthy foods available in countries across the region. Inspiration for the recipes in this cookbook mainly comes from the following Mediterranean countries.

EUROPEAN COUNTRIES	MIDDLE EASTERN COUNTRIES	NORTH AFRICAN COUNTRIES
Italy	Israel	Algeria
Greece	Lebanon	Libya
France	Turkey	Morocco
Spain	Syria	Egypt
Portugal		
Croatia		

Electric Pressure Cooker Sizes and Settings

Electric pressure cookers are available in a range of prices and sizes, suitable to meet most budget and batch-cooking needs. The average size you'll find most often is a 6-quart electric pressure cooker, which easily makes recipes with four to six servings. In some instances, such as beans, legumes, and grains, the 6-quart size can easily batch-cook a pound of the ingredient.

Smaller 3- to 4-quart electric pressure cookers are also widely available. These take up less counter space, but you will be limited in the amount of food that you can cook at one time. For those who like to cook large batches or regularly have more mouths to feed, the 8-quart electric pressure cookers can be a good choice. **For the purposes of this cookbook, all recipes were developed and tested using a 6-quart electric pressure cooker.**

There are a variety of universal settings found on electric pressure cookers. The following list provides additional information regarding the settings and instructions you will see in this cookbook:

- **SAUTÉ/BROWN:** Sautéing or browning some foods like meat and poultry or aromatics such as onions and garlic adds depth and flavor to the finished dish. This is not a pressure setting, so take care to not close the locking lid when using it.

- **ADDING LIQUID:** Liquid is integral to the pressure-cooking process since it essentially becomes the steam that creates pressure and cooks the food. Sufficient liquid is required if you want the electric pressure cooker to work properly.

- **LOCKING THE LID:** The way in which your lid locks in place will depend on the model, so be sure to follow the manufacturer's instructions. Generally speaking, you line up a specific part of the lid with a precise area on the pot and twist the lid into place. There is also a steam valve that should be set to sealed.

- **HIGH PRESSURE:** Generally, the high pressure setting registers at roughly 12 to 15 psi. The majority of recipes use the high pressure setting since it is most efficient. Please note that once you hit the high pressure button on the electric pressure cooker, it will take roughly 10 minutes to get up to pressure. This means that the timer will not activate until that happens. As such, all high pressure recipes in this cookbook account for an additional 10 minutes in the "total time."

- **LOW PRESSURE:** Generally, the low pressure setting registers at roughly 10 psi. The recipes that use low pressure usually require gentler cooking, such as fish, puddings, and certain egg dishes. Please note that once you hit the low pressure button on the electric pressure cooker, it will take roughly 5 minutes to get up to pressure. This means that the timer will not activate until that happens. As such, all low pressure recipes in this cookbook account for an additional 5 minutes in the "total time."

- **QUICK RELEASE:** Quick release is used when you want to stop the cooking process immediately or do not need to finish the recipe gently. To quick release, you release the steam valve from sealed to venting, which quickly and safely releases the steam that has built up in the pressure cooker.

- **NATURAL RELEASE:** Natural release is used when you want to allow the pressure to drop down naturally or finish the recipe gently. In this method, you turn off the electric pressure cooker, the steam valve remains closed, and the food continues to cook as the pressure dissipates over time. This can take anywhere from 15 minutes to 1 hour depending on the recipe. In some cases, you will use natural release for a certain amount of time, then finish with a quick release.

Electric Pressure Cooker Safety

New to the electric pressure cooker? No problem! As with any kitchen appliance, knowing how to safely use it is key. Luckily for us, modern electric pressure cookers are built with multiple safety features and are easier to use than ever before. The following safety tips will help get you started and keep you cooking safely and successfully.

TIP 1: Check the equipment. The rubber gasket, which is the ring of rubber that lines the cooker lid, should not be dried out or cracked. Checking to make sure the rim of the pot is clear of any dried food is also helpful to ensure that the seal cannot be broken during cooking.

TIP 2: Never "deep-fry" in your electric pressure cooker. Electric pressure cookers are meant to use liquid, such as water or broth, to create steam and pressure. Large amounts of oil can be dangerous and may cause the gasket to warp at high temperatures.

TIP 3: Use enough liquid, but do not overfill the inner pot. Enough liquid is required to create steam and maintain pressure. However, take care not to fill beyond the inner pot's "max line," or the pressure cooker may spit it out when you release pressure and open the lid after cooking. This is particularly true for foods that may froth or expand during cooking, such as grains and dried beans.

TIP 4: Release pressure safely. This is especially important for quick release! Make sure your face, hands, and body are away from the vent, or you could be burned by hot steam. Once pressure is fully released, the lid should easily twist. Never try to force it open.

TIP 5: Clean and store the cooker properly. This includes the inner pot as well as the lid and gasket. Store the lid upside down in the electric pressure cooker versus locked in place as well.

TIP 6: Run an initial water test. To do this, place 3 cups of water in the electric pressure cooker, close the lid, turn the steam release valve to the "sealed" position, and select high pressure for 5 minutes. Once the cooking time is complete, move the steam release valve to the "venting" position, and quick release the steam.

Helpful Accessories

You can absolutely use your electric pressure cooker to make delicious meals without buying any supplementary accessories. There are, however, some useful tools that may be a helpful and fun addition to your pressure cooker repertoire.

SILICONE MINI MITTS: These heat-resistant mitts protect your hands from steam, and the silicone allows you to easily grip the inner pot, steam racks, or bowls and safely lift them out.

TONGS: Tongs are a very helpful tool for reaching into the pot and turning or tossing ingredients. A variety of types are available, but silicone or stainless steel generally works best.

WIRE METAL STEAM RACK: This should come with your electric pressure cooker, but you may want to purchase an extra steam rack or stackable steam racks. It has arms that are used to place foods in or lift foods out of the pot. The steam rack is often used to keep foods directly off the bottom of the inner pot. Be sure to wear heat-resistant mitts when touching the rack immediately after cooking.

CLEANING AND CARING FOR YOUR COOKER

Electric pressure cookers are amazing appliances and a breeze to clean! Follow these tips to make sure you're keeping all the different parts clean and in tip-top shape.

1. WASH IT OUT IMMEDIATELY.
The inner pot should be removed and filled with hot, soapy water immediately after use.

2. SOAK IF NECESSARY.
The inner pot may be soaked if necessary and scrubbed as you would any other pot.

3. WIPE DOWN THE OUTSIDE.
Use a paper towel or microfiber cloth spritzed with distilled white vinegar to wipe down the outer casing of the cooker.

4. CLEAN THE RIM.
Get a cotton swab, foam paint brush, or straw with a cotton ball or paper towel attached to the end, dip it in distilled white vinegar, then run it around the rim of the pressure cooker to clean it out.

5. CLEAN THE SEALING RING.
This does not need to be done every time you use the pressure cooker, but the frequency may depend on how often you use the quick release function and whether or not you cook sticky or pungent foods. Detach the sealing ring from the lid, then run it through the dishwasher. Alternatively, you can add 2 cups of distilled white vinegar and some lemon zest to the inner pot, close and seal the lid, pressure cook on low for 2 minutes, and quick release.

STEAMER BASKET: This handy accessory is available in wire mesh, silicone, or expandable metal and is used to steam vegetables.

SILICONE EGG BITES MOLD: These stackable silicone molds allow you to make fun treats like egg bites! You can also use them for other bite-size recipes.

RAMEKINS: A set of 1-cup or 4-ounce ramekins is ideal for coddled eggs and individual desserts.

LOAF PAN: This is a great tool if you want to make meatloaf, quick bread, or cake recipes in your electric pressure cooker.

Tips and Troubleshooting

Dealing with issues that come up while using an electric pressure cooker is different than using conventional cooking methods. Because you cannot take off the lid "for a peek" or have any idea of what's really happening during the pressure-cooking process, you may encounter some issues after the dish is done cooking. The following is a list of common problems that may arise and solutions to help solve them.

PROBLEM: Scorching

SOLUTION: Scorching is often the result of not adding enough liquid. Be sure to follow the recipe, and use adequate liquid.

PROBLEM: Overcooked food

SOLUTION: Never let the electric pressure cooker switch to the "keep warm" setting. For quick release recipes, release the pressure immediately once the pressurized time is done. For natural release recipes, turn off the pressure cooker immediately once the pressurized time is done, then allow it to naturally release for the required amount of time as indicated in the recipe.

PROBLEM: Uneven cooking

SOLUTION: Follow the recipe, and prep the ingredients as directed.

PROBLEM: Undercooked food

SOLUTION: If you open the lid and find that the food is undercooked, simply hit the sauté button, and simmer the food until cooked through. You can also transfer the contents to a stovetop pot and gently simmer there, adding liquid as needed.

PROBLEM: Sauce is too thin or too thick

SOLUTION: If the sauce is thinner than you like, simply hit the sauté button, and simmer until it thickens to your liking. If the sauce is too thick, add more water or broth until it reaches your desired consistency.

PROBLEM: Cooking at high altitude

SOLUTION: At high altitudes, liquids evaporate faster and boil at lower temperatures compared to sea level. Most manufacturers include instructions regarding how to adjust cooking time. However, the general rule is to increase cooking time by 5 percent for every 1,000 feet you are located more than 2,000 feet above sea level. For example, if you are 4,000 feet above sea level and the cooking time is 30 minutes, you would increase that by 10 percent to 33 minutes. You may also have to add slightly more liquid to compensate for the additional time.

CHAPTER TWO

THE MEDITERRANEAN KITCHEN

A Mediterranean Meal

The typical Mediterranean diet offers plenty of animal-based lean protein options such as fish, eggs, and low-fat dairy, to name a few. It is a plant-based approach, but it is not a specifically vegan or vegetarian diet; however, you can easily take a Mediterranean approach if you follow either of those diets.

Mediterranean recipes are renowned for their simple cooking techniques and use of locally sourced whole foods. A variety of spices and herbs work together seamlessly to create flavor, texture, and healthy, delicious meals. Mediterranean meals may vary widely. Dinner could be a bowl filled with hummus and sautéed greens and vegetables topped with toasted nuts, or it may be a piece of roasted fish topped with pesto and served with braised lentils and tomatoes. As an overall lifestyle, the Mediterranean diet is easy to adhere to, with more and more people following it every year.

The Mediterranean diet is best summed up in the following diagram.

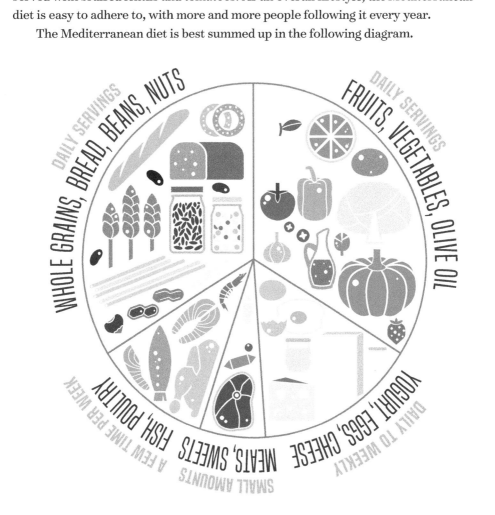

Plant-Based Powerhouses

The bulk of the Mediterranean diet is made up of vegetables, fruits, beans, legumes, and whole grains; these are the lifeblood of the Mediterranean kitchen. When prepared and cooked in the electric pressure cooker, these plant-based powerhouses shine. Beans, legumes, and grains in particular are superstars when it comes to pressure cooking.

Vegetables and Fruits

Fruits and vegetables are the workhorses of the Mediterranean diet. Full of vitamins, minerals, and antioxidants, these nutrient dynamos help power our day. Fruits and vegetables are inherently fiber-rich foods, which help us feel full, support decreased blood pressure, assist with weight management, and fend off inflammation and a variety of chronic diseases. Eat a variety of fruits and vegetables every day, from berries to bananas, garlic, onion, broccoli, and cauliflower—all of these will boost your mental and physical health.

- **SERVINGS:** Aim to consume five to seven servings of vegetables and three to four servings of fruit daily. One serving equates to ½ cup of fruit or vegetables or 1 cup of raw leafy greens. Trying to add a fruit or vegetable to every meal or snack is a great way to get you there!

- **ELECTRIC PRESSURE COOKER TIPS:** Most fruits and vegetables can be cooked in the electric pressure cooker. However, some are delicate and cook quickly, so many fruit and vegetable recipes utilize a quick release method.

Beans and Legumes

These plant-based protein sources include a variety of types, such as cannellini, kidney, and pinto beans; lentils; and soybeans. They are low in fat and high in fiber, complex carbohydrates, and protein, and they are a breeze to make in the electric pressure cooker from their dried state. Other key nutrients found in beans and legumes include iron, magnesium, and folate.

- **SERVINGS:** Aim for at least three servings of beans or legumes every week. One serving is ½ cup of cooked beans or legumes. Eating beans or legumes as a side dish or adding them to a salad or grain is an easy way to get them into your week in a delicious way.

- **ELECTRIC PRESSURE COOKER TIPS:** Soaking beans for 8 to 24 hours prior to cooking helps cut down the total cooking time. Some people choose to soak their dried beans prior to cooking them in the electric pressure cooker. However, the whole point of the pressure cooker (in my mind anyway) is to cut down on steps and overplanning, so the bean recipes you find in this cookbook will not require soaking overnight ahead of time.

Whole Grains and Starchy Vegetables

Whole grains and starchy vegetables are a good source of fiber, which helps slow the absorption of glucose in the blood. Packed with nutrients, these foods should be chosen over refined or processed carbohydrates whenever possible. Starchy vegetables include potatoes and sweet potatoes; whole grains include brown rice, farro, barley, oats, and whole-grain pasta.

- **SERVINGS:** Aim for four to six servings daily. One serving equates to ½ cup of cooked grains, 1 slice of whole-grain bread, or 1 medium sweet potato.

- **ELECTRIC PRESSURE COOKER TIPS:** Whole grains do very well in the electric pressure cooker, so they are quick and delicious. However, the moisture content in the individual grains may vary so they may get tender at different times. But never fear! If you open the lid after the cooking time ends and find your whole grains a bit too "al dente," simply lock the lid back in place, and leave them for a few minutes to steam.

Healthy Animal Proteins

The Mediterranean diet places a heavier emphasis on fish and seafood, with smaller portions of eggs, low-fat dairy, and lean cuts of poultry and meat. Overall, you are aiming for 6 ounces of protein from the following list on a daily basis. Quick-cooking cuts of seafood, meat, and poultry that are typically cooked on the stove or grill, such as sole, filet mignon, and chicken cutlets, are generally not appropriate cuts for the electric pressure cooker. Because they are lean with less fat and cartilage than other cuts, they may become rubbery or tough in a high-pressure cooking environment.

Seafood

Seafood, ranging from fish like salmon and cod to shellfish such as clams, mussels, and shrimp, are strongly emphasized and encouraged on the Mediterranean diet. Packed with lean protein, seafood is a powerhouse that also provides a variety of nutrients such as omega-3 fatty acids, zinc, and iron. Research shows that omega-3 fatty acids can help reduce inflammation and may help lower the risk of chronic diseases such as heart disease, cancer, and arthritis.

- **SERVINGS:** Aim for two to three servings of seafood on a weekly basis. One serving is 3 ounces, which is roughly the size of a deck of playing cards.

- **ELECTRIC PRESSURE COOKER TIPS:** Cooking fish and shellfish in an electric pressure cooker requires precise timing and attention to detail. However, I love that the cooker can be a great tool to create a flavorful sauce that is then used as the poaching liquid for the seafood.

Poultry

Poultry includes chicken, turkey, and duck, all of which can be found in a variety of cuts. Poultry is an excellent source of protein and provides a range of vitamins and minerals, including B vitamins, selenium, and choline.

- **SERVINGS:** Poultry should be eaten in moderation. One to two servings of poultry can be eaten on a weekly basis. One serving is 3 ounces, which is roughly the size of a deck of playing cards.

- **ELECTRIC PRESSURE COOKER TIPS:** The electric pressure cooker generally works very well with a variety of poultry. Cuts of poultry that have minimal fat, such as boneless, skinless chicken breast, simply need to be cooked with enough liquid to ensure tender, moist, flavorful results.

Eggs

Eggs are a great way to incorporate healthy animal proteins into your diet. One large egg provides 13 essential vitamins and minerals and 6 grams of high-quality protein. Eggs are particularly beneficial for those who do not eat poultry or meat.

- **SERVINGS:** Eggs should be eaten in moderation. One to two large eggs can be eaten three to four times per week.

- **ELECTRIC PRESSURE COOKER TIPS:** The electric pressure cooker works very well for specific types of egg cookery, such as soft- or hard-boiled, which you will see in this book. Eggs generally won't cook any faster compared to conventional methods, but peeling a hard-boiled egg made in the pressure cooker versus the stovetop will convince you it's worthwhile!

Dairy

Dairy foods, including yogurt and cheese, are recommended in moderate amounts in the Mediterranean diet. They are good sources of lean protein and a variety of vitamins and minerals. The dairy group provides essential nutrients such as calcium and potassium.

- **SERVINGS:** Aim to consume at least one serving of low-fat dairy daily. One serving equates to 1 cup of plain yogurt or Greek yogurt. Full-fat dairy, such as cheese, should be eaten in moderation, or two to three servings on a weekly basis. One serving of cheese equates to 1½ ounces.

- **ELECTRIC PRESSURE COOKER TIPS:** Dairy, like milk or cream, breaks under pressure unless it is part of a batter. As such, any recipes using these ingredients will typically add them at the end after the pressure-cooking time has ended.

Red Meat

Red meat, such as beef, pork, and lamb, can be part of the Mediterranean diet, especially lean, unprocessed cuts of meat. In just 3 ounces, red meat such as beef provides 10 essential nutrients, including protein, vitamin B_{12}, zinc, iron, and selenium.

- **SERVINGS:** Keep red meat to one to two servings on a weekly basis. One serving is 3 ounces, which is roughly the size of a deck of playing cards.

- **ELECTRIC PRESSURE COOKER TIPS:** The electric pressure cooker is an amazing appliance when it comes to tougher cuts of meat that are typically braised and take hours to cook conventionally, such as brisket, chuck roast, veal shanks, or lamb shoulder, to name a few. Using the electric pressure cooker cuts down on cooking time significantly, seals in flavor, and creates tender, tasty results.

SEAFOOD AND THE PRESSURE COOKER

Pressure cooking seafood can be a great way to get a healthy, delicious meal on the table in minimal time. However, fish and shellfish do require more attention and precise timing to avoid overcooking and becoming tough or rubbery. When preparing seafood, be sure to follow the specific time, pressure, and cooking guidelines in the recipe.

- Some shellfish, such as mussels or clams, can typically be added to the pressure cooker and steamed or cooked on low for a short time.
- Other shellfish, like shrimp, often taste best when added to the pressure cooker after a sauce has been made and they are simply sautéed in the inner pot after the sauce has completed its pressure-cooking time.
- Heartier fish, including salmon, tuna, monkfish, and cod, purchased in fillets, as a whole fish, or as a side of fish, work beautifully in the electric pressure cooker.

The Mediterranean Pantry

Getting your Mediterranean pantry together does not require a lot of difficult-to-find or expensive ingredients. Many of these essentials are likely to be in your home already! To get started, take a look at your pantry, refrigerator, and freezer and the following lists to make sure you have everything you may need.

Oils

Olive oil is a staple in the Mediterranean diet and the principal source of fat used for cooking, baking, and dressings. It is known for its heart-healthy monounsaturated fat content and anti-inflammatory properties. Olive oil will be your main go-to oil. Regular olive oil typically has a milder flavor and is best for all-purpose cooking. Extra-virgin olive oil can be used for some cooking, but it has a lower smoke point and a more fruity, tangy, or bold flavor that can truly shine as a finishing oil or as part of dressings, dips, or sauces. For a more neutral flavor, canola, avocado, and sunflower oil can be used. Oil should be stored tightly closed in a cool, dark place.

Nuts and Seeds

Nuts and seeds are good sources of healthy fats, plant-based protein, dietary fiber, and a variety of other nutrients. A study in the *American Journal of Clinical Nutrition* found that people who ate three servings of nuts on a weekly basis had lower indications of inflammation. The Mediterranean diet uses a wide variety of nuts and seeds, but in this book you will most often see almonds, walnuts, pine nuts, and pistachios.

Nuts and seeds are delicious as snacks, but they are also a great addition to many recipes to enhance the flavor, texture, and nutrition of a dish. In general, nuts and seeds are best stored in airtight containers in the refrigerator or freezer due to their high oil content.

Spices and Herbs

Herbs and spices are used to season or add flavor to dishes, which reduces the amount of salt necessary while you are cooking. Herbs used in cooking are typically leaves and stems, and spices are derived from bark, fruit, seeds, or other parts of trees or shrubs. For example, nutmeg is a seed and cinnamon is bark. It is truly amazing what herbs and spices can do. Taken on their own, potatoes may taste fairly bland; but add some tarragon and black pepper, and you have a whole new experience.

You will likely be familiar with many of the Mediterranean herbs and spices in this book, such as parsley, basil, and mint. However, I have included some that may be new to you.

- **ZA'ATAR** is a spice mixture of dried thyme, sesame seeds, and sumac. You can easily mix your own Za'atar spice blend if you like.

- **SUMAC** is a dried and ground spice that is typically dark red and has a citrus flavor.

- **HARISSA** is a chili paste or red pepper paste that is most often found in ready-made glass jars or tubes. It is often found in the international aisle of your grocery store but is also readily available online.

TO PRESSURE COOK OR NOT TO PRESSURE COOK?

Most foods can be cooked in the electric pressure cooker, but that does not mean they should be! Not all foods are destined for pressure cooker greatness.

The dishes and foods that typically work best are those that typically take long periods of time to cook with conventional methods. For example, tough cuts of meat, homemade stock, and dried beans are all great choices for pressure cooking. With the right recipe and precise timing, the electric pressure cooker is also a great appliance for cooking seafood and more delicate fruits and vegetables.

On the other hand, there are some foods that are best made conventionally. Pasta is one of these, and it can be very tricky to pressure cook, with a tendency to overcook and turn mushy. The same goes for anything that is delicate or meant to be crispy. Pressure cookers add moisture, so these types of foods may end up a soggy mess.

Indulging the Mediterranean Way

The Mediterranean diet is a lifestyle. Moderation and approaching food in a healthy, balanced way are main focal points. It also encourages fostering community and making meals social occasions. As such, savoring meals among family and friends can include enjoying an occasional glass or two of wine or a reasonable portion of dessert. As always, moderation is the key component.

- **WINE:** Making meals a social occasion is part of the Mediterranean lifestyle. One serving is 5 ounces, and having a few glasses per week is reasonable.

- **ADDED SUGAR:** Sometimes adding sugar to a dish is essential, as we will see in some of the dessert recipes. Added sugar is about 7 grams per serving. Limit yourself to five servings of added sugar per week.

The Book's Recipes

For me, part of the joy of cooking is creating recipes for others to enjoy and being able to experiment and try new things. And guess what? Experimenting in the kitchen can help build your cooking knowledge and confidence, too! This section will introduce you to the recipes to come, including the meanings of the labels, tips, and electric pressure cooker timing instructions.

Labels

To help you identify recipes that cater to specific dietary needs, look for the following labels.

DAIRY-FREE: Recipes that are free of cow's milk dairy products.

GLUTEN-FREE: Recipes that are free of gluten. Be sure to check the ingredient labels for items such as oats to ensure they are processed in a gluten-free facility.

Cook, Release, and Total Times

The following is a brief explanation of each time-related part of a recipe as it relates to electric pressure cooking time.

PREP TIME: This is the amount of active time spent to prep ingredients, such as chopping, peeling, and slicing.

PRESSURE COOK: This is the amount of active pressure cooking time.

RELEASE: Quick release will not add any time, but natural release will be indicated here with a specific amount of time.

TOTAL TIME: This is the total time to complete the entire recipe and encompasses prep time, sauté time, pressure cook time, simmering time, release time, and an additional 5 or 10 minutes to get to either low or high pressure.

Recipe Tips

The following tips are meant to help navigate the electric pressure cooker, the Mediterranean diet, and the recipes themselves.

HELPFUL HACK: Offers tips or tricks to make the prep, cooking process, or recipe easier or more efficient.

SIMPLE SWAP: Highlights ingredients that may be swapped out for a variety of reasons, such as allergies or to change up the flavor profile.

TROUBLESHOOTING TIP: Addresses potential electric pressure cooker issues that may pertain to that recipe.

SAVE FOR LATER: Suggestions for storing or freezing leftovers.

Let's get pressure cooking!

CHAPTER THREE

BREAKFAST

SAVORY STRATA Page 30

ALMOND BUTTER OATMEAL

Steel-cut oats are my favorite! They are made by running whole oats through a steel mill, which chops them into small pieces. This process creates a chewier texture with a nutty, hearty flavor. Oats are a great source of complex carbohydrates, dietary fiber, plant-based protein, and iron—perfect to get you going in the morning. I've paired these oats with almond butter and dried apricots, but feel free to swap them out for your favorite nut or seed butter and dried fruit.

3¾ cups water

1¼ cups steel-cut oats

½ cup almond butter

½ cup chopped dried apricots

SERVES 6

DAIRY-FREE, GLUTEN-FREE

Prep Time: 5 minutes

Pressure Cook: 10 to 13 minutes

Pressure Level: High

Release: 10 minutes Natural, then Quick

Total Time: 35 to 40 minutes

1. In the electric pressure cooker, combine the water and oats. Stir well. Secure the lid, and cook on high pressure for 10 minutes. (For creamier oats, cook on high pressure for 13 minutes.)

2. After cooking, let the pressure release naturally for 10 minutes, then quick release the remaining pressure. Unlock and remove the lid.

3. Stir in the almond butter and apricots. Serve warm.

SAVE FOR LATER: Transfer the cooked oats to a storage container, and let cool for 20 minutes. Cover and refrigerate for up to 1 week. To reheat, scoop out individual servings of the cooked oats. Add 1 tablespoon water or milk to the chilled oats. Reheat in either a small pot over medium-low heat or the microwave for about 2 minutes. Then add the almond butter and dried apricots.

PER SERVING: Calories: 290; Fat: 13g; Carbohydrates: 35g; Fiber: 6g; Sugar: 10g; Protein: 10g; Sodium: 6mg

EGG BITES

With such simple ingredients, these egg bites are a cinch to pull together. This recipe features asparagus, goat cheese, and chives. Egg bites can be stored in the refrigerator for 3 days and are great on-the-go, convenient breakfasts and snacks. I love making egg bites on a busy weekday morning, and my family loves having something nourishing on their way out the door.

6 large eggs

¼ cup reduced fat milk

2 asparagus spears, thinly sliced

⅓ cup crumbled goat cheese

2 tablespoons chopped fresh chives

½ teaspoon kosher salt

¼ teaspoon freshly ground black pepper

1. In a medium bowl, beat together the eggs and milk.

2. Stir in the asparagus, goat cheese, chives, salt, and pepper.

3. Ladle or pour the mixture into a 6-bite egg mold, and place it on a steam rack.

4. Cover the egg mold tightly with aluminum foil.

5. Pour 1 cup of water into the electric pressure cooker, then carefully place the steam rack and egg mold in the pot. Secure the lid, and cook on high pressure for 8 minutes.

6. After cooking, let the pressure release naturally for 5 minutes, then quick release the remaining pressure. Unlock and remove the lid.

7. Carefully remove the steam rack and egg mold. Using a spatula or fork, pop the egg bites out of the mold. Serve warm or at room temperature.

SERVES 3

GLUTEN-FREE

Prep Time: 10 minutes

Pressure Cook: 8 minutes

Pressure Level: High

Release: 5 minutes Natural, then Quick

Total Time: 30 to 35 minutes

SIMPLE SWAP: Egg bites are a super versatile breakfast option. Feel free to swap out the asparagus, goat cheese, and chives for whatever vegetables, cheese, and herbs you like! You can also make this dairy-free by using plant-based milk and removing the cheese entirely.

PER SERVING: Calories: 180; Fat: 12g; Carbohydrates: 2g; Fiber: 0g; Sugar: 2g; Protein: 15g; Sodium: 380mg

EGG SALAD WITH AVOCADO

Avocado has long been a staple in the Mediterranean diet. With healthy fats and a ton of fiber, this plant-based treasure is a natural fit. So why add eggs to your avocado toast? Protein! One large egg has 6 grams of protein and a lot of other great nutrients, including choline, vitamin B$_{12}$, and biotin. Together, they're a perfect combination.

1 ripe avocado, pitted, peeled, and diced

4 Hard-Boiled Eggs (page 144), peeled and chopped

⅓ cup chopped fresh dill

⅓ cup chopped fresh parsley

⅓ cup chopped fresh chives

Juice of 1 lemon

½ teaspoon kosher salt

¼ teaspoon freshly ground black pepper

4 whole-wheat or sourdough bread slices, toasted

SERVES 4

DAIRY-FREE

Prep Time: 15 minutes

Total Time: 15 minutes

HELPFUL HACK: Use an egg slicer to quickly chop the eggs. Simply place 1 hard-boiled egg in an egg slicer and slice through. Then turn the egg 90 degrees and slice through the other way.

PER SERVING: Calories: 235; Fat: 11g; Carbohydrates: 24g; Fiber: 4g; Sugar: 4g; Protein: 11g; Sodium: 380mg

1. In a medium bowl, mash the avocado.

2. Add the eggs, dill, parsley, chives, lemon juice, salt, and pepper. Mix together, keeping a chunky consistency.

3. Serve the egg salad with the toasted bread.

YOGURT PARFAIT

This scrumptious dish calls for plain yogurt that can be made in the electric pressure cooker. However, plain regular or Greek yogurt purchased at your local grocery store works just as well! Instead of buying a flavored yogurt, plain yogurt with fruit and natural sweeteners like honey are a great way to boost flavor and nutrients without all the added sugar. Warming spices like cinnamon, nutmeg, and ginger are also a great addition to this delightful breakfast treat.

2 cups Plain Yogurt (page 145) or store-bought plain yogurt

1 cup fresh or frozen blueberries

1 teaspoon honey

¼ cup sliced almonds

¼ cup shelled pistachios

2 mint sprigs (optional)

SERVES 2

GLUTEN-FREE

Prep Time: 10 minutes

Total Time: 10 minutes

1. In a medium bowl, mash together the yogurt, blueberries, and honey.

2. In 2 small serving bowls or clear lowball glasses, layer the yogurt mixture, almonds, and pistachios in any order you like.

3. Garnish with the mint (if using).

SIMPLE SWAP: Use any berries you like or a mixture of several. If using strawberries, be sure to slice or dice them before mashing with the yogurt. Maple syrup is also a great option to sweeten the yogurt a bit in place of the honey; or opt for sugar-free and do not add any sweetener. To transform this into a delectable dessert, add some toasted coconut and chocolate shavings.

PER SERVING: Calories: 180; Fat: 8g; Carbohydrates: 19g; Fiber: 2g; Sugar: 14g; Protein: 9g; Sodium: 95mg

SAVORY STRATA

This Italian-inspired savory strata is easy to throw together before you go to bed. Simply place it in the electric pressure cooker the next day, and you've got a delicious one-pot dish that's perfect for overnight guests or weekend brunch. It's also a great way to use up some vegetables, cheese, or bread. Looking for something to do with that two- to three-day-old bread? Make a strata!

1 cup Vegetable Stock (page 148) or store-bought vegetable stock

4 large eggs

1½ teaspoons Italian seasoning

½ teaspoon kosher salt

¼ teaspoon freshly ground black pepper

¼ teaspoon red pepper flakes

4 cups cubed sourdough bread

1 bunch Swiss chard, stemmed, leaves chopped

⅓ cup oil-packed sun-dried tomatoes, chopped

⅓ cup grated Parmesan cheese

Olive oil cooking spray, for coating the soufflé dish

¼ cup chopped fresh parsley (optional)

SERVES 6

Prep Time: 15 minutes, plus 2 hours to chill

Pressure Cook: 25 minutes

Pressure Level: High

Release: 10 minutes Natural, then Quick

Total Time: 1 hour, plus 2 hours to chill

SIMPLE SWAP: Feel free to swap out the Swiss chard and Parmesan for whatever leafy greens and cheese you like! Spinach or kale would work beautifully and pairs nicely with feta, goat cheese, or a variety of hard cheeses like Cheddar or Manchego.

PER SERVING: Calories: 270; Fat: 6g; Carbohydrates: 40g; Fiber: 2g; Sugar: 2g; Protein: 14g; Sodium: 700mg

1. In a large bowl, beat together the stock, eggs, Italian seasoning, salt, pepper, and red pepper flakes.

2. Mix in the bread, chard, tomatoes, and cheese. Cover, and refrigerate for 2 hours or up to overnight.

3. Lightly spray a 2-quart soufflé dish or 7-cup round glass container with cooking spray.

4. Transfer the egg mixture to the dish, cover tightly with aluminum foil, and place on a steam rack.

5. Pour 1½ cups of water into the electric pressure cooker, then carefully place the steam rack and dish in the pot. Secure the lid, and cook on high pressure for 25 minutes.

6. After cooking, let the pressure release naturally for 10 minutes, then quick release the remaining pressure. Unlock and remove the lid.

7. Carefully remove the steam rack and dish.

8. Garnish with the parsley (if using), and serve.

ZUCCHINI FRITTATA

This frittata is more like an egg casserole when prepared in the electric pressure cooker, but it is still delicious no matter what you call it. I love the combination of zucchini and feta, and the nutmeg adds a little something special to the mix. Feel free to use whole milk in place of the reduced fat milk, but do not swap out the cow's milk for plant-based milk, which will be too thin and produce a different result.

8 large eggs

⅓ cup reduced fat milk

½ teaspoon dried thyme

½ teaspoon kosher salt

¼ teaspoon freshly ground black pepper

¼ teaspoon ground nutmeg

1 cup grated zucchini (1 large)

⅓ cup crumbled feta cheese

Olive oil cooking spray, for coating the soufflé dish

SERVES 4

GLUTEN-FREE

Prep Time: 10 minutes

Pressure Cook: 25 minutes

Pressure Level: Low

Release: Quick

Total Time: 40 minutes

SIMPLE SWAP: Yellow squash or another vegetable you like may be swapped in for the zucchini. However, be sure to grate it so that the cooking time and water content stays the same.

PER SERVING: Calories: 185; Fat: 12g; Carbohydrates: 2g; Fiber: 1g; Sugar: 2g; Protein: 15g; Sodium: 400mg

1. In a large bowl, beat together the eggs, milk, thyme, salt, pepper, and nutmeg.

2. Mix in the zucchini and cheese.

3. Lightly spray a 2-quart soufflé dish or 7-cup round glass container with cooking spray.

4. Transfer the egg mixture to the dish, cover tightly with aluminum foil, and place on a steam rack.

5. Pour 1½ cups of water into the electric pressure cooker, then carefully place the steam rack and dish in the pot. Secure the lid, and cook on low pressure for 25 minutes.

6. After cooking, quick release the pressure. Unlock and remove the lid.

7. Carefully remove the steam rack, and serve.

CODDLED EGGS WITH SPINACH

Poached eggs are a much-loved breakfast or brunch favorite, but the electric pressure cooker is not the appliance to use. Next best thing? Coddled eggs! I love the look and taste of these individual servings of coddled eggs. They're steamed in perfect portions; serve these eggs with a side of crusty bread to mop up the yolk.

Olive oil cooking spray, for coating the ramekins

1 cup chopped baby spinach

¼ cup grated Parmesan cheese

2 teaspoons Za'atar

½ teaspoon kosher salt

½ teaspoon freshly ground black pepper

4 large eggs

1. Lightly spray 4 ramekins with cooking spray.

2. Divide the spinach, cheese, Za'atar, salt, and pepper equally among the ramekins.

3. Crack 1 egg into each ramekin, cover tightly with aluminum foil, and place on a steam rack. (The ramekins may need to be stacked slightly, but be sure not to stack them so that one completely covers another.)

4. Pour 1 cup of water into the electric pressure cooker, then carefully place the steam rack and ramekins in the pot. Secure the lid, and cook on low pressure for 4 minutes.

5. After cooking, quick release the pressure. Unlock and remove the lid.

6. Carefully remove the steam rack and ramekins. Serve immediately.

SERVES 4

GLUTEN-FREE

Prep Time: 10 minutes

Pressure Cook: 4 minutes

Pressure Level: Low

Release: Quick

Total Time: 20 minutes

SIMPLE SWAP: Coddled eggs will taste great with a range of mix-ins. Try chopped Swiss chard with Manchego or grated summer squash with goat cheese. You can also skip the mix-ins altogether and just cook the eggs on their own with some spices and a teaspoon of whole milk or cream for some richness.

PER SERVING: Calories: 100; Fat: 7g; Carbohydrates: 1g; Fiber: 0g; Sugar: 0g; Protein: 9g; Sodium: 315mg

CHAPTER FOUR

VEGETABLES AND SIDES

GREEN BEANS WITH CHRAIMEH SAUCE
Page 40

ARTICHOKES WITH YOGURT AÏOLI

Artichokes—abundant in Greece, Spain, France, and Italy—may seem intimidating but are easy to prepare in the electric pressure cooker. Once cooked, the outer leaves can be pulled off and enjoyed by gently using your teeth to scrape off the buttery underside of the leaves. Beyond the outer leaves, you'll want to remove the purple-topped inner leaves and the fuzzy inner choke that sits on top of the heart. (Eat the artichoke heart—it's the best part!)

FOR THE ARTICHOKES

2 large artichokes

FOR THE AÏOLI

½ cup Plain Yogurt (page 145) or store-bought plain yogurt

2 tablespoons chopped fresh chives

1 teaspoon freshly squeezed lemon juice

1 teaspoon Dijon mustard

1 garlic clove, grated

¼ teaspoon kosher salt

⅛ teaspoon freshly ground black pepper

SERVES 2

GLUTEN-FREE

Prep Time: 5 minutes

Pressure Cook: 8 minutes

Pressure Level: High

Release: Quick

Total Time: 20 to 25 minutes

TROUBLESHOOTING TIP: If the artichokes are large and crowd together or do not fit side by side, you can cook them one at a time. Or if you have a tall trivet designed for the electric pressure cooker, you can stack them. Simply set 1 artichoke on the steam rack, place the trivet in the pot over the first artichoke, then set the second artichoke on the trivet.

PER SERVING: Calories: 125; Fat: 1g; Carbohydrates: 23g; Fiber: 9g; Sugar: 6g; Protein: 9g; Sodium: 260mg

TO MAKE THE ARTICHOKES

1. Using kitchen shears, cut off the stem of the artichokes, and trim about 1 inch off the tip and the spiky outer leaves.

2. Pour 1 cup of water into the electric pressure cooker, and place a steam rack inside.

3. Place the artichokes on the steam rack. Secure the lid, and cook on high pressure for 8 minutes.

4. After cooking, quick release the pressure. Unlock and remove the lid.

TO MAKE THE AÏOLI

5. While the artichokes are cooking, in a small bowl, whisk together the yogurt, chives, lemon juice, mustard, garlic, salt, and pepper. Refrigerate until the artichokes are ready to eat.

6. Serve the artichokes with the aïoli on the side for dipping.

BRAISED FENNEL

Fennel is native to the Mediterranean, growing wild throughout many countries in the region. It is easy to spot with its thick stalks, feathery green leaves, and bright-yellow flowers. Raw fennel is reminiscent of celery in its texture and like licorice or anise in its taste, but when cooked, the flavor mellows out and the fennel bulb becomes silky. Pair this with the Shrimp with Lentils (page 92) for a well-rounded meal.

1 teaspoon extra-virgin olive oil

2 onions, quartered

2 fennel bulbs, trimmed, cored, and cut ½-inch thick; reserve and chop some fennel fronds for garnish

½ cup Vegetable Stock (page 148) or store-bought vegetable stock

1 teaspoon grated orange zest

½ cup freshly squeezed orange juice

¾ teaspoon kosher salt

SERVES 4

DAIRY-FREE, GLUTEN-FREE

Prep Time: 10 minutes

Pressure Cook: 3 minutes

Pressure Level: High

Release: Quick

Total Time: 30 to 35 minutes

1. Press the sauté button on the electric pressure cooker, allow it to heat up, then add the oil.

2. Add the onions, and sauté, turning once, for about 3 minutes, or until browned. Press the cancel button to stop cooking.

3. Add the fennel, stock, orange zest, orange juice, and salt. Mix together. Secure the lid, and cook on high pressure for 3 minutes.

4. After cooking, quick release the pressure. Unlock and remove the lid.

5. Press the sauté button, and cook for about 5 minutes, reducing the liquid to the desired thickness. Press the cancel button to stop cooking.

6. Garnish with chopped fennel fronds, and serve.

SIMPLE SWAP: The orange juice pairs beautifully with the fennel. If you don't have any oranges, bottled orange juice works well, or you can swap out the orange zest and juice for that of another citrus fruit like grapefruit or lemon.

PER SERVING: Calories: 80; Fat: 1g; Carbohydrates: 16g; Fiber: 5g; Sugar: 8g; Protein: 2g; Sodium: 290mg

EGGPLANT, SUMMER SQUASH, AND TOMATOES

This recipe is a variation of the French dish ratatouille. Try this recipe with any variety of eggplant or summer squash. Top this dish with toasted nuts or cheese, and serve over Basic Brown Rice (page 142) for a vegetarian meal.

1 teaspoon extra-virgin olive oil

1 eggplant, diced (1 pound)

2 summer squash, diced (1 pound)

1 onion, diced

2 garlic cloves, minced

1 (14½-ounce) can low-sodium diced tomatoes

½ cup water, Vegetable Stock (page 148), or store-bought vegetable stock

2 tablespoons freshly squeezed lemon juice

2 teaspoons dried oregano

2 teaspoons Italian seasoning

¾ teaspoon kosher salt

⅛ teaspoon freshly ground black pepper

1 bay leaf

SERVES 4

DAIRY-FREE, GLUTEN-FREE

Prep Time: 15 minutes

Pressure Cook: 4 minutes

Pressure Level: High

Release: Quick

Total Time: 30 to 35 minutes

SAVE FOR LATER: This recipe is easily batched up and saved for a future meal. Put the leftovers into containers, and refrigerate for up to 5 days or freeze for up to 3 months.

PER SERVING: Calories: 100; Fat: 2g; Carbohydrates: 19g; Fiber: 6g; Sugar: 12g; Protein: 4g; Sodium: 250mg

1. Press the sauté button on the electric pressure cooker, allow it to heat up, then add the oil.

2. Add the eggplant, squash, and onion. Sauté for about 3 minutes, or until softened.

3. Add the garlic, and sauté for 30 seconds, or until fragrant.

4. Add the tomatoes with their juices, water, lemon juice, oregano, Italian seasoning, salt, pepper, and bay leaf. Mix well. Press the cancel button to stop cooking.

5. Secure the lid, and cook on high pressure for 4 minutes.

6. After cooking, quick release the pressure. Unlock and remove the lid. Serve warm.

GREEN BEANS WITH CHRAIMEH SAUCE

I first came across Chraimeh sauce at a Libyan restaurant many years ago and have been making different versions of it ever since. Though it has roots in North Africa and Libya, variations can be found throughout the Mediterranean region. Traditionally, it is very spicy and often served with fish. My version is more mellow, but if you'd like to kick up the heat, add some cayenne and swap out the sweet paprika for hot or smoked paprika. In addition to green beans, Chraimeh sauce is delicious paired with other vegetables, meat, poultry, fish, or some crusty bread.

1 tablespoon avocado oil

5 garlic cloves, sliced

1 tablespoon caraway seeds

1 tablespoon ground cumin

2 teaspoons sweet paprika

1 teaspoon ground cinnamon

3 tablespoons tomato paste

Juice of 1 lime

2 teaspoons honey

1 teaspoon kosher salt

1 cup water

1 pound green beans, trimmed

SERVES 4

DAIRY-FREE, GLUTEN-FREE

Prep Time: 15 minutes

Pressure Cook: 1 minute

Pressure Level: Low

Release: Quick

Total Time: 20 to 25 minutes

HELPFUL HACK: To speed up prep time, purchase green beans or haricots verts that have already been cleaned and trimmed.

PER SERVING: Calories: 95; Fat: 4g; Carbohydrates: 15g; Fiber: 4g; Sugar: 9g; Protein: 3g; Sodium: 325mg

1. Press the sauté button on the electric pressure cooker, allow it to heat up, then add the oil.

2. Add the garlic, caraway seeds, cumin, paprika, and cinnamon. Sauté for about 1 minute, or until fragrant.

3. Add the tomato paste, lime juice, honey, and salt. Sauté for 30 seconds.

4. Add the water, and mix well.

5. Add the green beans, and mix together. Press the cancel button to stop cooking.

6. Secure the lid, and cook on low pressure for 1 minute.

7. After cooking, quick release the pressure. Unlock and remove the lid.

8. Pour the green beans and sauce into a serving dish, and serve immediately or at room temperature.

POTATOES WITH GREENS

There are many different varieties of potatoes, but I find that small, waxy types work best in this dish. This is because they are less starchy and retain their shape and structure better in the electric pressure cooker. Look for mini or small potatoes that are one bite when cut in half. Waxy potato varieties include new potatoes, red bliss, fingerlings, and blue or red potatoes, to name a few. Other hearty greens, such as collard greens or mustard greens, can be used in place of the kale if preferred.

1 teaspoon extra-virgin olive oil

5 garlic cloves, sliced

2 bunches kale, stemmed and chopped

1½ pounds small new potatoes, halved

1 cup water, Vegetable Stock (page 148), or store-bought vegetable stock

2 tablespoons freshly squeezed lemon juice

1 teaspoon kosher salt

¼ teaspoon freshly ground black pepper

SERVES 4

DAIRY-FREE, GLUTEN-FREE

Prep Time: 15 minutes

Pressure Cook: 7 minutes

Pressure Level: High

Release: Quick

Total Time: 30 to 35 minutes

HELPFUL HACK: Pre-chopped kale can be used to cut down on prep time.

PER SERVING: Calories: 180; Fat: 2g; Carbohydrates: 39g; Fiber: 7g; Sugar: 6g; Protein: 9g; Sodium: 320mg

1. Press the sauté button on the electric pressure cooker, allow it to heat up, then add the oil.

2. Add the garlic, and sauté for about 30 seconds, or until fragrant.

3. Add the kale, potatoes, water, lemon juice, salt, and pepper. Mix well. Press the cancel button to stop cooking.

4. Secure the lid, and cook on high pressure for 7 minutes.

5. After cooking, quick release the pressure. Unlock and remove the lid. Serve warm.

BEETS WITH TAHINI YOGURT

Beets are delicious, nutritious, and easy to make in the electric pressure cooker. Wild beets originated in northern Africa and Europe along the Mediterranean Sea. These earthy root vegetables can be found in a range of colors, including purple, pink, golden, white, and red-and-white striped. And be sure to save those beet greens; they'll work beautifully in the Savory Strata (page 30).

FOR THE BEETS

1 pound beets, trimmed

FOR THE TAHINI YOGURT

½ cup Plain Yogurt (page 145) or store-bought plain yogurt

⅓ cup tahini

2 tablespoons freshly squeezed lemon juice

2 tablespoons water

¾ teaspoon kosher salt

½ teaspoon maple syrup

¼ teaspoon ground cumin

⅛ teaspoon cayenne pepper

SERVES 4

GLUTEN-FREE

Prep Time: 15 minutes
Pressure Cook: 20 minutes
Pressure Level: High
Release: Quick
Total Time: 55 minutes

SAVE FOR LATER: The tahini yogurt is easily batched up and saved for a future meal, and it tastes great on top of vegetables, meat, poultry, or as a dip for pita. Put the leftovers into a container, and refrigerate for up to 5 days.

PER SERVING: Calories: 210; Fat: 12g; Carbohydrates: 19g; Fiber: 5g; Sugar: 13g; Protein: 9g; Sodium: 390mg

TO MAKE THE BEETS

1. Fill a bowl with ice water.

2. Pour 1 cup of water into the electric pressure cooker. Place the beets in a steamer basket or on a steam rack in the pot. Secure the lid, and cook on high pressure for 20 minutes.

3. After cooking, quick release the pressure. Unlock and remove the lid.

4. Transfer the beets to the ice water bath, and let cool for 10 minutes.

5. Peel the beets by gently rubbing them with your fingers to remove the peel. Cut into quarters or rounds.

TO MAKE THE TAHINI YOGURT

6. While the beets are cooking, in a small mixing bowl, whisk together the yogurt, tahini, lemon juice, water, salt, maple syrup, cumin, and cayenne. Refrigerate until the beets are ready to eat.

7. Serve the beets topped with the tahini yogurt, or serve with the yogurt on the side for dipping.

SMASHED POTATOES

Is there anything better than potatoes that are crispy on the outside and tender on the inside? This recipe is a delight and a crowd-pleaser for sure. Don't let the double cooking methods deter you, it's well worth it and still a cinch to prepare! Pair with the Lamb Meatloaf with Tahini Sauce (page 114) and a fresh salad for a delicious, well-balanced meal.

1½ pounds mini potatoes

2 tablespoons extra-virgin olive oil

1 teaspoon kosher salt

¼ teaspoon freshly ground black pepper

6 rosemary sprigs

SERVES 4

DAIRY-FREE, GLUTEN-FREE

Prep Time: 5 minutes
Pressure Cook: 15 minutes
Pressure Level: High
Release: Quick
Total Time: 55 minutes

1. Pour 1 cup of water into the electric pressure cooker. Place the potatoes in a steamer basket in the pot. Secure the lid, and cook on high pressure for 15 minutes.

2. Preheat the oven to 450°F. Line a baking sheet with aluminum foil or parchment paper.

3. After cooking, quick release the pressure. Unlock and remove the lid.

4. Put the potatoes on the prepared baking sheet, and toss with the oil, salt, and pepper.

5. Spread the potatoes out on the baking sheet in a single layer, then using the bottom of a glass or measuring cup, flatten or smash them.

6. Place the rosemary sprigs on the baking sheet.

7. Transfer the baking sheet to the oven, and roast for 25 minutes, or until the potatoes are golden brown. Remove from the oven. Serve immediately.

SIMPLE SWAP: Change up the herbs and spices here however you like. Toss the potatoes with cayenne, garlic powder, and onion powder in place of the salt and pepper, or use crushed garlic cloves instead of—or in addition to—the rosemary.

PER SERVING: Calories: 175; Fat: 7g; Carbohydrates: 29g; Fiber: 3g; Sugar: 3g; Protein: 5g; Sodium: 280mg

CREAMY POLENTA WITH CRÈME FRAÎCHE

Polenta is a classic Italian side dish that is made from cooked cornmeal or corn grits. For this recipe, look for polenta labeled "coarse-ground." It should also be labeled as either "yellow polenta" or "corn grits." A widespread belief is that polenta takes a lot of time and whisking to be cooked properly, but the electric pressure cooker makes it easy. Serve it as a side dish, or use it in place of pasta. Eggplant, Summer Squash, and Tomatoes (page 39) would be a perfect topper for the creamy polenta!

4 cups Vegetable Stock (page 148) or store-bought vegetable stock

3 tablespoons unsalted butter, cubed

½ teaspoon kosher salt

1 cup coarse-ground yellow polenta or corn grits

½ cup grated Pecorino Romano cheese

⅓ cup crème fraîche

¼ teaspoon freshly ground black pepper

SERVES 6

GLUTEN-FREE

Prep Time: 10 minutes

Pressure Cook: 8 minutes

Pressure Level: High

Release: 20 minutes Natural, then Quick

Total Time: 55 minutes

SIMPLE SWAP: Can't find crème fraîche? Mascarpone cheese, cream cheese, or sour cream can be used instead.

PER SERVING: Calories: 225; Fat: 15g; Carbohydrates: 20g; Fiber: 3g; Sugar: 1g; Protein: 6g; Sodium: 320mg

1. In the electric pressure cooker, combine the stock, butter, and salt. Press the sauté button. Melt the butter, and simmer for about 5 minutes.

2. Stir in the polenta, and whisk constantly for 2 minutes. Press the cancel button to stop cooking.

3. Secure the lid, and cook on high pressure for 8 minutes.

4. After cooking, let the pressure release naturally for 20 minutes, then quick release the remaining pressure. Unlock and remove the lid.

5. Stir in the cheese, crème fraîche, and pepper. Continue to stir together for about 1 minute, or until the cheese has melted and the polenta smooths out a bit. Transfer to a serving dish.

BEAN SALAD

A simple salad with a variety of fresh vegetables, beans, and a delicious dressing is a fantastic light lunch or part of a larger meal. The vegetables provide a range of vitamins and minerals, the beans are an excellent source of plant-based protein, and the tahini dressing is chock-full of healthy fats. To add even more protein, fiber, and tasty crunch, garnish the salad with some toasted walnuts or almonds.

2 cups Basic Chickpeas (page 143) or canned chickpeas

½ cup Tahini Dressing (page 151)

1 pint cherry tomatoes, halved

2 carrots, diced

1 hothouse cucumber, diced

1 red bell pepper, diced

2 celery stalks, diced

SERVES 4

DAIRY-FREE, GLUTEN-FREE

Prep Time: 20 minutes

Total Time: 20 minutes

SIMPLE SWAP: Although this recipe calls for cooked chickpeas, also known as garbanzo beans, any beans you like can be used. A variety of vegetables would also work well in this fresh salad.

PER SERVING: Calories: 340; Fat: 20g; Carbohydrates: 32g; Fiber: 9g; Sugar: 9g; Protein: 10g; Sodium: 335mg

1. In a large bowl, combine the chickpeas and tahini dressing. Mix well.

2. Add the tomatoes, carrots, cucumber, bell pepper, and celery. Toss together well, and serve.

SMASHED FAVA BEANS WITH TOAST

Fava beans, also known as broad beans, are native to North Africa and the Mediterranean region and are used in a variety of recipes. They take some time and care to prepare since they must be soaked and peeled but are well worth it. If you see fresh fava beans at your local farmer's market, they can be swapped in and used in this recipe. If using fresh fava beans, you do not need to soak them overnight.

1 pound dried fava beans

8 cups water

½ cup minced fresh mint leaves

3 tablespoons extra-virgin olive oil

Grated zest of 1 lemon

Juice of 1 lemon

½ teaspoon kosher salt

½ teaspoon red pepper flakes

½ cup grated Parmesan cheese

12 whole-wheat or sourdough bread slices, toasted

SERVES 6

Prep Time: 1 hour, plus overnight to soak

Pressure Cook: 7 minutes

Pressure Level: Low

Release: 15 minutes Natural, then Quick

Total Time: 1 hour 30 minutes, plus overnight to soak

SIMPLE SWAP: Don't want to spend the extra time soaking and peeling, or can't find fava beans? Use dried soybeans or frozen shelled edamame instead.

PER SERVING: Calories: 370; Fat: 14g; Carbohydrates: 50g; Fiber: 9g; Sugar: 6g; Protein: 16g; Sodium: 620mg

1. Put the fava beans in the electric pressure cooker, fill with water, then refrigerate overnight or for up to 24 hours.

2. Drain and rinse the beans. Peel the outer skin off each bean.

3. In the electric pressure cooker, combine the beans and 8 cups of water. Secure the lid, and cook on low pressure for 7 minutes.

4. While the beans are cooking, in a large bowl, mix together the mint, oil, lemon zest, lemon juice, salt, and red pepper flakes.

5. After cooking, let the pressure release naturally for 15 minutes, then quick release the remaining pressure. Unlock and remove the lid. Drain the beans.

6. Add the beans and cheese to the mint mixture. Mix well, and smash to your desired consistency.

7. Serve the smashed beans with the toasted bread.

FARRO WITH HERBY YOGURT

Farro is a popular grain throughout Italy. It is a distant cousin of wheat but looks like a jumbo-size grain of brown rice with a flat, cleaved belly and a rounded back. It has a rich, earthy, nutty flavor that pairs beautifully with this herby yogurt. Farro is an excellent source of fiber, plant-based protein, complex carbohydrates, and a range of vitamins and minerals. Pair this dish with a side salad or some roasted vegetables for a delicious vegetarian meal.

FOR THE FARRO

3 cups water

1 cup farro

FOR THE HERBY YOGURT

1 cup fresh mint leaves

1 cup fresh parsley

⅓ cup buttermilk

Grated zest of 1 lemon

2 tablespoons freshly squeezed lemon juice

1 teaspoon kosher salt

¼ teaspoon freshly ground black pepper

⅔ cup Plain Yogurt (page 145) or store-bought plain yogurt

SERVES 4

GLUTEN-FREE

Prep Time: 5 minutes
Pressure Cook: 25 minutes
Pressure Level: High
Release: 10 minutes
Natural, then Quick
Total Time: 50 minutes

SAVE FOR LATER: If you want to save some plain farro to use later, allow it to cool, then transfer to an airtight container and refrigerate for up to 1 week, or freeze for up to 3 months.

PER SERVING: Calories: 215; Fat: 1g; Carbohydrates: 39g; Fiber: 4g; Sugar: 4g; Protein: 10g; Sodium: 390mg

TO MAKE THE FARRO

1. In the electric pressure cooker, combine the water and farro. Secure the lid, and cook on high pressure for 25 minutes.

2. After cooking, let the pressure release naturally for 10 minutes, then quick release the remaining pressure. Unlock and remove the lid. Drain the farro.

TO MAKE THE HERBY YOGURT

3. While the farro is cooking, in a blender, combine the mint, parsley, buttermilk, lemon zest, lemon juice, salt, and pepper. Puree, then pour into a bowl.

4. Add the yogurt, and whisk together. Refrigerate until the farro is cooked.

5. Add the farro to the yogurt mixture, and stir together well. Serve immediately warm, at room temperature, or cold.

GREEK-STYLE LENTILS

Lentils are an excellent source of plant-based protein and iron, making them a perfect alternative to meat. They are a rich source of many vitamins and minerals, including B vitamins, magnesium, zinc, and potassium, as well as dietary fiber. There are dozens of lentil varieties, ranging from black to yellow, red, and green. For this recipe, I prefer green, or French, lentils because they hold their shape well and do not turn mushy in the electric pressure cooker.

1 tablespoon extra-virgin olive oil

1 onion, finely diced

2 carrots, finely diced

2 celery stalks, finely diced

1 teaspoon kosher salt

2 garlic cloves, minced

1 tablespoon tomato paste

1 teaspoon dried oregano

½ teaspoon ground cinnamon

⅛ teaspoon red pepper flakes

2½ cups Vegetable Stock (page 148) or store-bought vegetable stock

1½ cups dried French green lentils, picked through and rinsed

1 (14½-ounce) can low-sodium diced tomatoes

SERVES 6

DAIRY-FREE, GLUTEN-FREE

Prep Time: 15 minutes

Pressure Cook: 20 minutes

Pressure Level: High

Release: 10 minutes Natural, then Quick

Total Time: 1 hour 5 minutes

SIMPLE SWAP: If you have fresh tomatoes, you can chop about 2 cups and use them in place of the canned tomatoes. If you use raw tomatoes, sauté them in step 2 and add an extra ½ cup of stock in step 5.

PER SERVING: Calories: 235; Fat: 3g; Carbohydrates: 38g; Fiber: 17g; Sugar: 6g; Protein: 14g; Sodium: 287mg

1. Press the sauté button on the electric pressure cooker, allow it to heat up, then add the oil.

2. Add the onion, carrots, celery, and salt. Sauté, stirring frequently, for 5 minutes, or until softened.

3. Add the garlic, and sauté for 30 seconds, or until fragrant.

4. Add the tomato paste, oregano, cinnamon, and red pepper flakes. Sauté for 30 seconds.

5. Add the stock, lentils, and tomatoes with their juices. Mix together. Press the cancel button to stop cooking.

6. Secure the lid, and cook on high pressure for 20 minutes.

7. After cooking, let the pressure release naturally for 10 minutes, then quick release the remaining pressure. Unlock and remove the lid.

8. Stir the lentil mixture well, and serve.

CHAPTER FIVE

MEATLESS MAINS

MOROCCAN TAGINE WITH BUTTERNUT
SQUASH AND CHICKPEAS Page 68

BEAN SOUP

Beans are one of the most common foods eaten worldwide, thanks to their affordability and versatility. My recipe uses kidney beans, but any beans you like will work well and taste great; you can also try a mix of different types of beans or use a "bean soup mix." Beans are an excellent source of plant-based protein, dietary fiber, folate, iron, and magnesium.

1 teaspoon extra-virgin olive oil

1 onion, diced

2 celery stalks, diced

2 carrots, diced

4 cups water

4 cups Vegetable Stock (page 148) or store-bought vegetable stock

1 pound dried kidney beans

1 tablespoon dried parsley

1 tablespoon dried oregano

1 teaspoon dried thyme

2 bay leaves

1 (14½-ounce) can low-sodium diced tomatoes

3 tablespoons freshly squeezed lemon juice

1 teaspoon kosher salt

¼ teaspoon freshly ground black pepper

SERVES 10

DAIRY-FREE, GLUTEN-FREE

Prep Time: 15 minutes

Pressure Cook: 45 minutes

Pressure Level: High

Release: 20 minutes Natural, then Quick

Total Time: 1 hour 40 minutes

SAVE FOR LATER: Portion out the soup into containers, label each container with the name and date, then freeze for up to 6 months.

PER SERVING: Calories: 185; Fat: 1g; Carbohydrates: 33g; Fiber: 13g; Sugar: 4g; Protein: 11g; Sodium: 200mg

1. Press the sauté button on the electric pressure cooker, allow it to heat up for 1 minute, then add the oil.

2. Add the onion, celery, and carrots. Sauté, stirring frequently, for 5 minutes, or until softened.

3. Add the water, stock, beans, parsley, oregano, thyme, and bay leaves. Press the cancel button to stop cooking.

4. Secure the lid, and cook on high pressure for 45 minutes.

5. After cooking, let the pressure release naturally for 20 minutes, then quick release the remaining pressure. Unlock and remove the lid.

6. Mix in the tomatoes with their juices, lemon juice, salt, and pepper.

7. Mash some of the beans to thicken, if desired, and serve warm.

SPICED CHICKPEA BOWLS

These spiced chickpea bowls make for an easy, delicious lunch or light dinner. And if you're looking to shave some minutes off the prep time, pull out that food processor. That handy-dandy kitchen appliance can get those carrots grated and that fennel sliced in no time.

FOR THE YOGURT

1 cup Plain Yogurt (page 145) or store-bought plain yogurt

2 tablespoons freshly squeezed lemon juice

½ teaspoon kosher salt

½ teaspoon ground cumin

¼ teaspoon ground coriander

FOR THE BOWLS

3 cups Basic Chickpeas (page 143) or canned chickpeas

2 carrots, grated

1 fennel bulb, sliced

1 ripe avocado, pitted, peeled, and sliced

¼ cup chopped fresh cilantro

¼ cup chopped fresh parsley

SERVES 4

GLUTEN-FREE

Prep Time: 15 minutes

Total Time: 15 minutes

SIMPLE SWAP: If you don't have cooked chickpeas, the canned variety can be used. The chickpeas can also be swapped out for lentils or other beans you like.

PER SERVING: Calories: 330; Fat: 9g; Carbohydrates: 49g; Fiber: 14g; Sugar: 14g; Protein: 16g; Sodium: 250mg

TO MAKE THE YOGURT

1. In a small bowl, mix together the yogurt, lemon juice, salt, cumin, and coriander.

TO MAKE THE BOWLS

2. Divide the yogurt mixture among 4 serving bowls.

3. Divide the chickpeas, carrots, and fennel among the bowls on top of the yogurt.

4. Divide the avocado, and put on top of each serving bowl.

5. Serve the bowls garnished with the cilantro and parsley.

RIBOLLITA

Ribollita, which means "reboiled" in Italian, is a Tuscan vegetable soup that is thickened with bread. It is a delicious way to stretch bread out over a week by turning it into a vital part of this hearty stew. Feel free to throw in other vegetables you like or need to use up, including diced potatoes and kale or other greens.

3 tablespoons extra-virgin olive oil, divided

1 onion, diced

2 carrots, diced

2 celery stalks, diced

1 teaspoon kosher salt

6 garlic cloves, minced

¼ teaspoon freshly ground black pepper

¼ teaspoon red pepper flakes

4 cups Vegetable Stock (page 148) or store-bought vegetable stock

1 (28-ounce) can low-sodium diced tomatoes

1 cup dried cannellini beans

1 small Parmesan rind (optional)

2 rosemary sprigs, leaves chopped

½ loaf (8 ounces) day-old crusty bread, torn into 1- to 2-inch pieces

⅓ cup grated Parmesan cheese

SERVES 6

Prep Time: 20 minutes

Pressure Cook: 30 minutes

Pressure Level: High

Release: 20 minutes Natural, then Quick

Total Time: 1 hour 40 minutes

HELPFUL HACK: If you prefer to skip the oven entirely (steps 7 through 12), simply mix all the bread and Parmesan directly into the electric pressure cooker once step 4 is complete. This will not give you a crispy bread and cheese topping, but it will still taste delicious!

PER SERVING: Calories: 390; Fat: 10g; Carbohydrates: 58g; Fiber: 9g; Sugar: 10g; Protein: 16g; Sodium: 650mg

1. Press the sauté button on the electric pressure cooker, allow it to heat up for 1 minute, then add 2 tablespoons of oil.

2. Add the onion, carrots, celery, and salt. Sauté for 3 minutes, or until softened.

3. Add the garlic, pepper, and red pepper flakes. Sauté for 30 seconds, or until fragrant.

4. Add the stock, tomatoes with their juices, beans, Parmesan rind (if using), and rosemary. Mix well. Press the cancel button to stop cooking.

5. Secure the lid, and cook on high pressure for 30 minutes.

6. After cooking, let the pressure release naturally for 20 minutes, then quick release the remaining pressure. Unlock and remove the lid.

7. While the pressure releases, preheat the oven to 500°F.

8. Transfer the entire contents of the pot to a large, oven-safe Dutch oven or pot.

9. Mix in half of the bread, and stir together well.

10. Scatter the remaining bread across the top of the mixture in the pot.

11. Drizzle with the remaining 1 tablespoon of oil, and sprinkle with the cheese.

12. Transfer the pot to the oven, and cook for 15 minutes, or until the topping is golden brown. Remove from the oven. Serve immediately.

SILKEN TOMATO SOUP

Tofu, made from soybeans, is a popular plant-based protein. It contains high levels of minerals, such as calcium, potassium, magnesium, and iron, and other nutrients, including B vitamins and fiber. Because of its neutral taste, tofu easily absorbs other flavors, making it a versatile, nutrient-dense addition to any dish. Plant-based silken tofu can add creaminess without the cream to a variety of dishes like soups, smoothies, and desserts.

1 onion, diced

1 carrot, diced

1 tablespoon extra-virgin olive oil

1 teaspoon kosher salt

2 garlic cloves, minced

¼ teaspoon freshly ground black pepper

1 (28-ounce) can low-sodium whole tomatoes

2 cups Vegetable Stock (page 148) or store-bought vegetable stock

1 tablespoon honey

1 (16-ounce) package silken tofu

¼ cup fresh basil leaves, cut into ribbons

SERVES 6

DAIRY-FREE, GLUTEN-FREE

Prep Time: 20 minutes

Pressure Cook: 5 minutes

Pressure Level: High

Release: 10 minutes Natural, then Quick

Total Time: 45 to 50 minutes

SAVE FOR LATER: If planning to freeze the soup, put in airtight containers or resealable freezer bags after step 3. Do not add the silken tofu until planning to eat the soup.

PER SERVING: Calories: 115; Fat: 4g; Carbohydrates: 15g; Fiber: 3g; Sugar: 10g; Protein: 5g; Sodium: 345mg

1. Press the sauté button on the electric pressure cooker, allow it to heat up, then add the onions, carrot, oil, and salt. Sauté for 3 minutes, or until softened.

2. Add the garlic and pepper. Sauté for 30 seconds, or until fragrant.

3. Add the tomatoes with their juices, stock, and honey. Mix well. Press the cancel button to stop cooking.

4. Secure the lid, and cook on high pressure for 5 minutes.

5. After cooking, let the pressure release naturally for 10 minutes, then quick release the remaining pressure. Unlock and remove the lid.

6. Add the tofu, and using an immersion blender, puree the contents of the inner pot until smooth. (If you don't have an immersion blender, transfer to a regular blender, and puree until smooth.)

7. Serve the soup garnished with the basil.

LENTIL AND EGGPLANT STEW

Eggplant belongs to the nightshade family, along with tomatoes and potatoes. The most popular variety of eggplant looks like a large, pear-shaped egg—get it, "eggplant"?—and has a glossy, deep-purple skin and a cream-colored flesh that has a spongy consistency when raw. There are several varieties of eggplant available, all of which will taste great in this dish.

1 red onion, diced

2 tablespoons extra-virgin olive oil

1 teaspoon kosher salt

2 tablespoons fresh thyme leaves

4 garlic cloves, sliced

¼ teaspoon freshly ground black pepper

1 eggplant, diced (1½ pounds)

1 pint cherry tomatoes

½ cup white wine

2 cups water

1 cup dried French green lentils

Juice of ½ lemon

Crème fraîche, for serving (optional)

SERVES 4

GLUTEN-FREE

Prep Time: 15 minutes

Pressure Cook: 15 minutes

Pressure Level: High

Release: 15 minutes Natural, then Quick

Total Time: 1 hour 5 minutes

HELPFUL HACK: Diced eggplant will cook faster and integrate into the final dish more than large chunks.

PER SERVING: Calories: 320; Fat: 8g; Carbohydrates: 45g; Fiber: 20g; Sugar: 9g; Protein: 15g; Sodium: 300mg

1. Press the sauté button on the electric pressure cooker, allow it to heat up, then add the onion, oil, and salt. Sauté for 3 minutes, or until the onion has softened.

2. Add the thyme, garlic, and pepper. Sauté for 30 seconds, or until fragrant.

3. Add the eggplant and tomatoes. Sauté for 3 minutes, or until softened.

4. Add the wine, and deglaze: mix well, scrape up any brown bits, and reduce the wine, for about 1 minute.

5. Add the water and lentils. Mix well. Press the cancel button to stop cooking.

6. Secure the lid, and cook on high pressure for 15 minutes.

7. After cooking, let the pressure release naturally for 15 minutes, then quick release the remaining pressure. Unlock and remove the lid.

8. Add the lemon juice, and mix well. If desired, press the sauté button, and cook, stirring occasionally, to thicken to the desired consistency.

9. Serve the stew garnished with a dollop of crème fraîche (if using).

MUJADARA

Mujadara is a popular plant-based protein-rich Middle Eastern dish known throughout Israel, Lebanon, and Egypt, to name a few. It is a variation of rice pilaf made with brown rice, lentils, and caramelized or crispy onions. I've paired this version with yogurt, but feel free to swap it out and top with a fried egg or roasted fish instead.

FOR THE RICE AND LENTILS

1 tablespoon extra-virgin olive oil

4 garlic cloves, smashed and peeled

2 teaspoons ground cumin

1 teaspoon ground coriander

3 cups Vegetable Stock (page 148) or store-bought vegetable stock

1 cup long-grain brown rice

1 cup dried French green lentils

1 teaspoon kosher salt

¼ teaspoon freshly ground black pepper

1 bay leaf

FOR THE MUJADARA

⅓ cup vegetable oil or canola oil

2 onions, julienned

½ cup chopped fresh parsley, divided

1 cup Plain Yogurt (page 145) or store-bought plain yogurt

Hot sauce, for serving (optional)

Tahini, for serving (optional)

SERVES 4

GLUTEN-FREE

Prep Time: 15 minutes

Pressure Cook: 16 minutes

Pressure Level: High

Release: 16 minutes Natural, then Quick

Total Time: 55 minutes to 1 hour

TROUBLESHOOTING TIP: The pressure cooking and release timing for this dish is based on long-grain brown rice. If you use a different variety, such as short-grain brown rice, the cooking time may change.

PER SERVING: Calories: 530; Fat: 16g; Carbohydrates: 77g; Fiber: 18g; Sugar: 10g; Protein: 20g; Sodium: 435mg

TO MAKE THE RICE AND LENTILS

1. Press the sauté button on the electric pressure cooker, allow it to heat up, then add the oil.

2. Add the garlic, cumin, and coriander. Sauté for 30 seconds, or until fragrant.

3. Add the stock, rice, lentils, salt, pepper, and bay leaf. Mix well. Press the cancel button to stop cooking.

4. Secure the lid, and cook on high pressure for 16 minutes.

5. After cooking, let the pressure release naturally for 16 minutes, then quick release the remaining pressure. Unlock and remove the lid.

6. Mix together the rice and lentils, remove the bay leaf, then place lid askew over the pot to partially cover.

TO MAKE THE MUJADARA

7. While the rice and lentils are cooking, in a large skillet, heat the oil over medium heat. Line a plate with paper towels.

8. Add the onions, and cook, stirring occasionally, for 30 minutes, or until golden and cooked to your desired crispness. Remove from the heat. Transfer to the prepared plate.

9. Mix half of the onions and ¼ cup of parsley in with the rice and lentils. Transfer to a large serving dish.

10. Serve the mujadara with the remaining onions, ¼ cup of parsley, the yogurt, hot sauce (if using), and tahini (if using) on the side.

VEGETABLE BOURGUIGNON

Meaty mushrooms are the highlight of this vegetarian spin on the classic French beef stew. Feel free to swap out the carrots and celery for parsnips, turnips, or rutabaga. If you're not concerned about keeping this vegetarian, beef stock is a great substitute for the vegetable stock. Serve this on its own or over Creamy Polenta with Crème Fraîche (page 45).

2 tablespoons extra-virgin olive oil

1 tablespoon unsalted butter

1½ pounds mixed mushrooms, such as cremini, white button, shiitake, sliced

2 celery stalks, diced

2 carrots, diced

1 leek, white and light green parts only, sliced

3 garlic cloves, minced

1 bay leaf

1 teaspoon dried thyme

1 teaspoon kosher salt

¼ teaspoon freshly ground black pepper

1 tablespoon tomato paste

1 tablespoon all-purpose flour

1½ cups red wine

1 (14-ounce bag) frozen pearl onions

1½ cups Vegetable Stock (page 148) or store-bought vegetable stock

1½ tablespoons soy sauce

½ cup chopped fresh parsley

SERVES 4

Prep Time: 20 minutes
Pressure Cook: 5 minutes
Pressure Level: High
Release: Quick
Total Time: 1 hour 10 minutes

SIMPLE SWAP: To make this dish gluten-free, swap out the all-purpose flour for gluten-free flour, and use gluten-free tamari in place of the soy sauce.

PER SERVING: Calories: 270; Fat: 10g; Carbohydrates: 27g; Fiber: 5g; Sugar: 11g; Protein: 7g; Sodium: 590mg

1. Press the sauté button on the electric pressure cooker, allow it to heat up, then add the oil and butter.

2. Once the butter has melted, add the mushrooms, celery, carrots, and leek. Sauté, stirring occasionally, for about 15 minutes, or until the mushrooms release most of their moisture.

3. Add the garlic, bay leaf, thyme, salt, and pepper. Cook for 5 minutes, or until fragrant. Try to boil off some of the water from cooking the mushrooms.

4. Add the tomato paste, and sauté for 1 minute.

5. Sprinkle the flour over the vegetables.

6. Add the wine, and deglaze: mix well, and scrape up any brown bits on the bottom of the pot. Reduce the wine by half, about 5 minutes.

7. Add the onions, stock, and soy sauce. Mix well. Press the cancel button to stop cooking.

8. Secure the lid, and cook on high pressure for 5 minutes.

9. After cooking, quick release the pressure. Unlock and remove the lid, then mix well.

10. Press the sauté button, and cook, stirring occasionally, until the desired consistency is reached. Press the cancel button to stop cooking.

11. Serve the stew garnished with the parsley.

RED LENTIL BURGERS

These plant-based burgers are beautifully golden with fragrant spices. Serve them on their own or topped with Plain Yogurt (page 145), spicy mango chutney, or a refreshing tomato-cucumber salad. I am partial to cashews for this recipe, but any nuts you like will be delicious.

1 tablespoon extra-virgin olive oil

1 onion, finely diced

1 red bell pepper, finely diced

1 tablespoon grated fresh ginger

1 tablespoon ground cumin

2 garlic cloves, minced

1 teaspoon ground coriander

1 teaspoon ground turmeric

1 teaspoon kosher salt

½ teaspoon ground cinnamon

¼ teaspoon freshly ground black pepper

1½ cups water

1 cup dried red lentils

2 cups Basic Brown Rice (page 142)

½ cup chopped toasted cashews

⅓ cup minced fresh cilantro

Juice of ½ lemon

SERVES 6
DAIRY-FREE, GLUTEN-FREE

Prep Time: 20 minutes
Pressure Cook: 3 minutes
Pressure Level: High
Release: 10 minutes Natural, then Quick
Total Time: 1 hour 20 minutes

SAVE FOR LATER: Put the leftover patties in resealable freezer bags, separated by pieces of parchment or wax paper. Be sure to label the bag with the name of the food and date. These patties should last up to 3 months in the freezer.

PER SERVING: Calories: 280; Fat: 8g; Carbohydrates: 41g; Fiber: 7g; Sugar: 3g; Protein: 13g; Sodium: 200mg

1. Press the sauté button on the electric pressure cooker, allow it to heat up, then add the oil.

2. Add the onion and bell pepper. Sauté for about 3 minutes, or until soft.

3. Add the ginger, cumin, garlic, coriander, turmeric, salt, cinnamon, and pepper. Sauté for 1 minute, or until fragrant.

4. Add the water and lentils. Mix well. Press the cancel button to stop cooking.

5. Secure the lid, and cook on high pressure for 3 minutes.

6. After cooking, let the pressure release naturally for 10 minutes, then quick release the remaining pressure. Unlock and remove the lid, then mix well.

7. Preheat the oven to 400°F. Line a baking sheet with parchment paper.

8. Carefully remove the inner pot, and put it on a trivet on the counter near the baking sheet.

9. Add the rice, cashews, cilantro, and lemon juice to the lentil mixture. Mix well. Spoon heaping ½-cup portions onto the prepared baking sheet. Using the bottom of the measuring cup or a glass, flatten them out slightly.

10. Transfer the baking sheet to the oven, and bake for 30 minutes, or until the patties are slightly golden brown. Remove from the oven. Serve immediately.

MOROCCAN TAGINE WITH BUTTERNUT SQUASH AND CHICKPEAS

Tagine is a stew-like dish that often contains meat, poultry, or fish and a variety of vegetables or fruit. My version is vegan and full of the plant-based protein powerhouse, chickpeas; a variety of vegetables; and aromatic Moroccan spices. If you like the idea of fruit in your tagine, add ½ cup of raisins or dried apricots in step 6. Serve over some Basic Brown Rice (page 142) or another grain, such as couscous, to soak up the delicious liquid.

1 tablespoon extra-virgin olive oil

1 onion, julienned

5 garlic cloves, minced

3 (2-inch) strips lemon zest

1 teaspoon ground cumin

¾ teaspoon kosher salt

½ teaspoon ground cinnamon

½ teaspoon ground coriander

⅛ teaspoon cayenne pepper

1 (1½-pound) butternut squash, peeled, seeded, and cut into 1-inch pieces

1 (14½-ounce) can low-sodium diced tomatoes

2 cups Vegetable Stock (page 148) or store-bought vegetable stock

1½ cups dried chickpeas, soaked for 8 hours or overnight

½ cup chopped pitted Kalamata olives

½ cup chopped fresh cilantro

Juice of ½ lemon

SERVES 6

DAIRY-FREE, GLUTEN-FREE

Prep Time: 20 minutes, plus 8 hours to soak

Pressure Cook: 25 minutes

Pressure Level: High

Release: Quick

Total Time: 1 hour 5 minutes, plus 8 hours to soak

HELPFUL HACK: Shave off some prep time by purchasing butternut squash already peeled, seeded, and cut into pieces.

PER SERVING: Calories: 300; Fat: 7g; Carbohydrates: 51g; Fiber: 13g; Sugar: 12g; Protein: 12g; Sodium: 391mg

1. Press the sauté button on the electric pressure cooker, allow it to heat up, then add the oil.

2. Add the onion, and sauté for about 2 minutes, or until softened.

3. Add the garlic, and sauté for 30 seconds, or until fragrant.

4. Add the lemon zest, cumin, salt, cinnamon, coriander, and cayenne. Sauté for 30 seconds, or until fragrant.

5. Add the squash and tomatoes with their juices. Mix well, and scrape up any brown bits on the bottom of the pot.

6. Add the stock and chickpeas. Mix well. Press the cancel button to stop cooking.

7. Secure the lid, and cook on high pressure for 25 minutes.

8. After cooking, quick release the pressure. Unlock and remove the lid, then mix well.

9. Press the sauté button, and cook for 5 minutes, reducing the liquid slightly.

10. Add the olives, cilantro, and lemon juice. Mix well. Press the cancel button to stop cooking. Serve immediately.

RISOTTO WITH MUSHROOMS AND ASPARAGUS

Risotto is a common Italian comfort food comprised of tender rice in a creamy sauce. There are a few short-grain varieties of rice that work best, but Arborio is my favorite. When making risotto, be sure to choose short-grain rice because the short, plump grains are best suited to absorb liquid, impart creaminess to the dish, maintain texture, and have a good bite.

1 tablespoon unsalted butter

1 tablespoon extra-virgin olive oil

8 ounces cremini mushrooms, thinly sliced

8 asparagus spears, thinly sliced

1 onion, finely diced

½ teaspoon kosher salt

¼ teaspoon freshly ground black pepper

3 tablespoons chopped fresh sage leaves

2 garlic cloves, minced

1½ cups Arborio rice

½ cup white wine

4 cups Vegetable Stock (page 148) or store-bought vegetable stock, warmed

½ cup grated Parmesan cheese

SERVES 4

GLUTEN-FREE

Prep Time: 20 minutes

Pressure Cook: 6 minutes

Pressure Level: High

Release: Quick

Total Time: 45 to 50 minutes

SIMPLE SWAP: Risotto is a super versatile vegetarian option. Feel free to swap out the asparagus, mushrooms, and sage for other vegetables and herbs you like! You can also make this dairy-free by removing the cheese and swapping the butter for oil.

PER SERVING: Calories: 480; Fat: 11g; Carbohydrates: 77g; Fiber: 4g; Sugar: 6g; Protein: 16g; Sodium: 470mg

1. Press the sauté button on the electric pressure cooker, allow it to heat up, then add the butter and oil.

2. Once the butter has melted, add the mushrooms, asparagus, onion, salt, and pepper. Sauté, stirring occasionally, for about 8 minutes, or until softened.

3. Add the sage and garlic. Sauté for 30 seconds, or until fragrant.

4. Add the rice, and sauté for 1 minute, or until starting to look translucent.

5. Add the wine, and deglaze: mix well, and scrape up any brown bits on the bottom of the pot. Reduce the wine by half, about 1 minute.

6. Add the stock, and mix well. Press the cancel button to stop cooking.

7. Secure the lid, and cook on high pressure for 6 minutes.

8. After cooking, quick release the pressure. Unlock and remove the lid, then mix the risotto well. If liquid still remains, press the sauté button, and cook, stirring continuously, until most of the liquid has been absorbed.

9. Add the cheese, and mix well. Press the cancel button to stop cooking. Serve immediately.

SPAGHETTI SQUASH WITH CHERRY TOMATOES, BASIL, AND FETA

Spaghetti squash is part of the winter squash family. It is typically large, yellow skinned, and oblong with a light-colored flesh that pulls away in strands resembling spaghetti when cooked. It is fairly neutral in flavor, has a tender and chewy texture, and is often used as a swap-in for pasta or grains. It is low in calories but is nutrient dense.

1½ cups water

1 (3- to 3½-pound) spaghetti squash, halved and seeded

2 pints cherry tomatoes, halved

½ cup crumbled feta cheese

2 tablespoons extra-virgin olive oil

2 tablespoons freshly squeezed lemon juice

½ teaspoon kosher salt

¼ teaspoon freshly ground black pepper

⅓ cup pine nuts, toasted

¼ cup fresh basil leaves, cut into ribbons (optional)

SERVES 4

GLUTEN-FREE

Prep Time: 15 minutes

Pressure Cook: 10 minutes

Pressure Level: High

Release: Quick

Total Time: 35 minutes

HELPFUL HACK: Sometimes large squash, such as spaghetti squash, can be difficult to cut in half. To make the job easier, simply put the squash in the microwave and cook in 30-second intervals until you are able to cut it in half.

PER SERVING: Calories: 500; Fat: 24g; Carbohydrates: 58g; Fiber: 16g; Sugar: 14g; Protein: 20g; Sodium: 350mg

1. Pour the water into the electric pressure cooker, then add the squash, skin-side down and angled so as not to completely cover one half with the other half. Secure the lid, and cook on high pressure for 10 minutes.

2. After cooking, quick release the pressure. Unlock and remove the lid.

3. Carefully transfer the squash to a cutting board. Using a fork, scrape the flesh out of the squash halves; it should come out easily and look similar to spaghetti.

4. In a large bowl, toss together the tomatoes, cheese, oil, lemon juice, salt, and pepper.

5. Add the squash strands to bowl, and toss.

6. Garnish with the pine nuts and basil (if using), and serve.

STUFFED SWEET POTATOES

Did you know there are more than 400 different varieties of sweet potatoes grown worldwide? They are all generally starchy and slightly sweet, but vary in shape, color, and texture, each with its own taste profile. They're all delicious and incredibly versatile, so grab your favorites and get these stuffed sweet potatoes going! A great addition to this dish is your favorite steamed or roasted vegetables.

4 medium (6- to 8-ounce) sweet potatoes

2 cups Basic Beans (page 143) or canned beans

1 cup Tzatziki (page 147)

SERVES 4
GLUTEN-FREE

Prep Time: 5 minutes
Pressure Cook: 12 minutes
Pressure Level: High
Release: Quick
Total Time: 25 to 30 minutes

1. Pour 1 cup of water into the electric pressure cooker, and place the steam rack in the pot. Place the sweet potatoes on the steam rack. Secure the lid, and cook on high pressure for 12 minutes.

2. After cooking, quick release the pressure. Unlock and remove the lid.

3. Carefully remove the sweet potatoes. Slice open lengthwise, and using a fork, fluff the inner flesh.

4. Stuff the sweet potatoes with the beans and tzatziki, and serve.

SAVE FOR LATER: Making sweet potatoes in the electric pressure cooker is a great way to meal prep for the week. They can be served as a hearty vegetarian main dish, as this recipe shows, but they can also be integrated in other ways throughout the week.

PER SERVING: Calories: 290; Fat: 5g; Carbohydrates: 52g; Fiber: 10g; Sugar: 11g; Protein: 12g; Sodium: 180mg

JAMMY EGGS WITH HUMMUS AND RICE SALAD

I love having a variety of flavors, textures, and types of food all in the same bowl. This delicious, simple dish provides all that you need in the form of creamy hummus, crisp greens, tender brown rice, and jammy soft-boiled eggs. For an extra boost of crunch, add your favorite toasted nuts as a topping. Perfect for a lunch break or light supper.

1½ cups Hummus (page 146) or store-bought hummus

2 cups Basic Brown Rice (page 142)

8 cups mixed greens, such as arugula, baby spinach, green or red leaf lettuce

4 Soft-Boiled Eggs (page 144), peeled and halved

SERVES 4

DAIRY-FREE, GLUTEN-FREE

Prep Time: 15 minutes
Total Time: 15 minutes

SIMPLE SWAP: Any type of whole grain will work well in this dish. Feel free to swap out the brown rice for quinoa, farro, or black rice.

PER SERVING: Calories: 375; Fat: 17g; Carbohydrates: 43g; Fiber: 8g; Sugar: 3g; Protein: 15g; Sodium: 290mg

1. Spoon and spread out the hummus along the bottom of a large serving platter.

2. Top with the rice.

3. Scatter the greens on top.

4. Place the eggs on top, and serve.

PASTA WITH MARINARA SAUCE

This quick weeknight pasta with homemade sauce is sure to be a crowd-pleaser. To guarantee that the pasta does not overcook, the pressure cooking time is only 5 minutes. After the pressure is released, there's another 5 minutes, which allows the rigatoni to reach perfect al dente doneness.

3 tablespoons extra-virgin olive oil

5 garlic cloves, sliced

1 (28-ounce) can low-sodium whole tomatoes, crushed with hands

1 tablespoon Italian seasoning

1 teaspoon honey

1 teaspoon kosher salt

¼ teaspoon freshly ground black pepper

1 pound rigatoni

2 cups Vegetable Stock (page 148) or store-bought vegetable stock

1½ cups water

½ cup grated Parmesan cheese

½ cup fresh basil leaves, cut into ribbons

SERVES 6

Prep Time: 10 minutes

Pressure Cook: 5 minutes

Pressure Level: High

Release: 5 minutes Natural, then Quick

Total Time: 40 to 45 minutes

SIMPLE SWAP: Any short, sturdy pasta will work in this recipe. Feel free to swap out the rigatoni for penne or ziti, for example.

PER SERVING: Calories: 415; Fat: 11g; Carbohydrates: 64g; Fiber: 4g; Sugar: 8g; Protein: 14g; Sodium: 375mg

1. Press the sauté button on the electric pressure cooker, allow it to heat up, then add the oil.

2. Add the garlic, and sauté for about 30 seconds, or until fragrant.

3. Add the tomatoes with their juices, Italian seasoning, honey, salt, and pepper. Mix well. Simmer for about 5 minutes, or until thickened.

4. Stir in the rigatoni, stock, and water. Mix well, making sure all the rigatoni is submerged. Press the cancel button to stop cooking.

5. Secure the lid, and cook on high pressure for 5 minutes.

6. After cooking, let the pressure release naturally for 5 minutes, then quick release the remaining pressure. Unlock and remove the lid, mix well, and let stand for 5 minutes.

7. Serve the pasta garnished with the cheese and basil.

LENTIL RAGÙ

Looking for a plant-based alternative to a traditional Bolognese sauce, also known as vegan Bolognese? Look no further than this lentil ragù! Whether you are a vegetarian or not, this dish is a great way to sneak some more vegetables into your day. Perfect for a Meatless Monday or, let's face it, delicious any day of the week, this sauce goes great with my Creamy Polenta with Crème Fraîche (page 45), or for an extra dose of veggies, serve it over zucchini noodles.

1 tablespoon extra-virgin olive oil

1 onion, diced

1 carrot, diced

1 teaspoon kosher salt

¼ teaspoon freshly ground black pepper

1 tablespoon dried basil

3 garlic cloves, minced

1 teaspoon dried thyme

1 teaspoon dried oregano

3 tablespoons tomato paste

3 cups Vegetable Stock (page 148) or store-bought vegetable stock

1 (15-ounce) can tomato sauce

1 (14½-ounce) can low-sodium diced tomatoes

1½ cups dried brown lentils

1 tablespoon red-wine vinegar

½ cup chopped fresh basil leaves

SERVES 6

GLUTEN-FREE

Prep Time: 10 minutes

Pressure Cook: 15 minutes

Pressure Level: High

Release: 15 minutes Natural, then Quick

Total Time: 55 minutes

SAVE FOR LATER: Put any leftovers into an airtight container, and freeze. I recommend using appropriate portion-size containers so that you can defrost smaller quantities if needed. Don't forget to label the containers with the dish name and date!

PER SERVING: Calories: 250; Fat: 3g; Carbohydrates: 42g; Fiber: 18g; Sugar: 9g; Protein: 14g; Sodium: 300mg

1. Press the sauté button on the electric pressure cooker, allow it to heat up, then add the oil.

2. Add the onion, carrot, salt, and pepper. Sauté for about 3 minutes, or until softened.

3. Add the basil, garlic, thyme, and oregano. Sauté for 30 seconds, or until fragrant.

4. Add the tomato paste, and sauté for 1 minute.

5. Add the stock, tomato sauce, tomatoes with their juices, and lentils. Mix well. Press the cancel button to stop cooking.

6. Secure the lid, and cook on high pressure for 15 minutes.

7. After cooking, let the pressure release naturally for 15 minutes, then quick release the remaining pressure. Unlock and remove the lid, and mix well.

8. Add the vinegar, and mix well.

9. Serve the ragù garnished with the basil.

COUSCOUS WITH EGGPLANT

Although couscous looks like a grain, it is actually a form of pasta. Couscous is made by rubbing semolina flour until tiny pieces are formed. Regular couscous is very small, whereas Israeli couscous is larger and similar to the size of a small pearl. This size gives more of a chewy bite to dishes compared to the smaller couscous variety.

1 tablespoon extra-virgin olive oil

1 onion, diced

1 tablespoon capers, drained and rinsed

2 garlic cloves, minced

½ teaspoon kosher salt

¼ teaspoon freshly ground black pepper

¼ teaspoon red pepper flakes

1 eggplant, diced (1 pound)

1 bunch kale, stemmed and chopped

2 cups Vegetable Stock (page 148) or store-bought vegetable stock

1¼ cups Israeli couscous

2 oregano sprigs, stemmed

2 thyme sprigs, stemmed

SERVES 4

DAIRY-FREE, GLUTEN-FREE

Prep Time: 20 minutes

Pressure Cook: 10 minutes

Pressure Level: High

Release: Quick

Total Time: 50 minutes to 1 hour

HELPFUL HACK: Be sure to dice the eggplant into ½- to 1-inch pieces and chop or tear the kale into small pieces. This will make it easier to cook and eat.

PER SERVING: Calories: 345; Fat: 5g; Carbohydrates: 71g; Fiber: 9g; Sugar: 10g; Protein: 14g; Sodium: 285mg

1. Press the sauté button on the electric pressure cooker, allow it to heat up, then add the oil.

2. Add the onion, and sauté for about 2 minutes, or until softened.

3. Add the capers, garlic, salt, pepper, and red pepper flakes. Sauté for about 30 seconds, or until fragrant.

4. Add the eggplant, and sauté for about 3 minutes, or until softened.

5. Add the kale, and cook, stirring, for about 1 minute, or until wilted.

6. Add the stock, couscous, oregano, and thyme. Mix together. Press the cancel button to stop cooking.

7. Secure the lid, and cook on high pressure for 10 minutes.

8. After cooking, quick release the pressure. Unlock and remove the lid, mix well, and let stand for 5 to 10 minutes. Serve warm.

CHAPTER SIX

SEAFOOD

MUSSELS WITH HARISSA Page 83

STEAMED CLAMS

Steamed clams are an easy, delicious dinner if you're in the mood for a pot of seafood. Clam shells can be fairly sandy, so be sure to scrub them well with a plastic brush prior to cooking. If any clam shells do not open after cooking, place the lid back on top askew, turn on the sauté function, and simmer for a few minutes until they open. If there are any remaining that do not open, discard them before serving.

2 pounds littleneck clams, washed and scrubbed

½ cup Vegetable Stock (page 148) or store-bought vegetable stock

½ cup white wine

2 tablespoons chopped fresh basil leaves

1 tablespoon extra-virgin olive oil

1 tablespoon freshly squeezed lemon juice

Crusty bread, for serving

SERVES 2

DAIRY-FREE, GLUTEN-FREE

Prep Time: 10 minutes

Pressure Cook: 4 minutes

Pressure Level: High

Release: 15 minutes Natural, then Quick

Total Time: 40 to 45 minutes

1. In the electric pressure cooker, combine the clams, stock, wine, basil, oil, and lemon juice. Secure the lid, and cook on high pressure for 4 minutes.

2. After cooking, let the pressure release naturally for 15 minutes, then quick release the remaining pressure. Unlock and remove the lid. If some clams are still closed, press the sauté button, and simmer for 1 to 2 minutes. Press the cancel button to stop cooking. Discard any unopened clams. Transfer to a serving dish.

3. Serve the clams with crusty bread.

SIMPLE SWAP: If you cannot find littleneck clams or simply prefer a different type, any clams will work well with this recipe.

PER SERVING: Calories: 340; Fat: 4g; Carbohydrates: 13g; Fiber: 1g; Sugar: 1g; Protein: 58g; Sodium: 320mg

MUSSELS WITH HARISSA

Have you tried harissa? It is a spicy, aromatic, and flavorful pepper or chili paste that is widely used in Mediterranean cooking. It may vary depending on the country, but it is generally a blend of hot chile peppers, olive oil, garlic, and spices. It may range from mild to hot, so be sure to choose whichever you prefer. It is most commonly found in ready-made jars, tubes, or cans in the grocery store.

2 tablespoons extra-virgin olive oil

1 shallot, diced

1 cup Vegetable Stock (page 148) or store-bought vegetable stock

1 tablespoon harissa

1 (14-ounce) can artichoke hearts, drained and rinsed

1 cup diced bell pepper

2 pounds mussels, scrubbed and debearded

2 tablespoons chopped fresh parsley

Crusty bread, for serving

SERVES 2

DAIRY-FREE, GLUTEN-FREE

Prep Time: 15 minutes
Pressure Cook: 2 minutes
Pressure Level: High
Release: Quick
Total Time: 30 minutes

TROUBLESHOOTING TIP: To clean mussels, put them in a colander in the sink under running water, and use a scrubbing brush to rub off any debris. Discard any mussels with open or cracked shells. To debeard, grab the fibers that may be sprouting from the shell, and pull off toward the hinge.

PER SERVING: Calories: 300; Fat: 12g; Carbohydrates: 16g; Fiber: 3g; Sugar: 3g; Protein: 29g; Sodium: 900mg

1. Press the sauté button on the electric pressure cooker, allow it to heat up, then add the oil.

2. Add the shallot, and sauté for 3 minutes, or until softened.

3. Add the stock and harissa. Deglaze: mix well, and scrape up any brown bits on the bottom of the pot.

4. Add the artichoke hearts and bell pepper. Mix well.

5. Add the mussels. Press the cancel button to stop cooking.

6. Secure the lid, and cook on high pressure for 2 minutes.

7. After cooking, quick release the pressure. Unlock and remove the lid.

8. Transfer the mussels to a large serving bowl.

9. Garnish with the parsley, and serve with crusty bread.

CIOPPINO

Cioppino is basically a type of seafood stew that can be found in Spain and the European area of the Mediterranean. There are many different variations, and all are tasty! I've bulked up this version with lots of vegetables, making it a hearty and healthy lunch or dinner. Be sure to have some pita bread or crusty bread to serve with it to soak up the delicious broth.

2 tablespoons extra-virgin olive oil

1 fennel bulb, cored and diced

1 onion, diced

1 carrot, diced

2 garlic cloves, sliced

1 teaspoon dried oregano

1 teaspoon dried thyme

¾ teaspoon kosher salt

¼ teaspoon red pepper flakes

½ cup white wine

1 (28-ounce) can low-sodium diced tomatoes

1 cup fish stock, Vegetable Stock (page 148), or store-bought vegetable stock

8 ounces skinless cod fillets, cut into 1-inch pieces

8 ounces calamari rings

8 ounces frozen shrimp, peeled and deveined

Crusty bread, for serving

SERVES 4

DAIRY-FREE, GLUTEN-FREE

Prep Time: 20 minutes
Pressure Cook: 1 minute
Pressure Level: Low
Release: Quick
Total Time: 30 to 35 minutes

SIMPLE SWAP: This recipe works well with any fish you like. Feel free to swap out the cod for whatever you prefer, including halibut or bass. Sea scallops also make a nice addition if you want to add those in place of the calamari or shrimp.

PER SERVING: Calories: 310; Fat: 9g; Carbohydrates: 23g; Fiber: 6g; Sugar: 12g; Protein: 30g; Sodium: 740mg

1. Press the sauté button on the electric pressure cooker, allow it to heat up, then add the oil.

2. Add the fennel, onion, and carrot. Sauté for 3 minutes, or until softened.

3. Add the garlic, oregano, thyme, salt, and red pepper flakes. Sauté for 30 seconds, or until fragrant.

4. Add the wine, and deglaze: mix well, and scrape up any brown bits on the bottom of the pot. Reduce the wine by half, about 3 minutes.

5. Add the tomatoes with their juices and the stock. Mix well.

6. Add the cod, calamari, and shrimp. Press the cancel button to stop cooking.

7. Secure the lid, and cook on low pressure for 1 minute.

8. After cooking, quick release the pressure. Unlock and remove the lid, then mix well.

9. Ladle the cioppino into bowls, and serve with crusty bread.

POACHED SHRIMP WITH MEDITERRANEAN "COCKTAIL SAUCE"

I love this recipe because it is super quick and uses shrimp straight from the freezer. For best results, choose peeled and deveined shrimp or EZ-peel shrimp that are large, so 31 to 40 per pound. The poached shrimp is meant to be served cold, but it will be just as delicious if you skip the ice bath in step 4 and serve it warm.

FOR THE SHRIMP

1 pound frozen shrimp

2 cups water

1 teaspoon kosher salt

FOR THE COCKTAIL SAUCE

¼ cup water

¼ cup harissa

¼ cup chopped fresh mint leaves

Juice of ½ lemon

SERVES 4

DAIRY-FREE, GLUTEN-FREE

Prep Time: 5 minutes

Pressure Cook: 1 minute

Pressure Level: Low

Release: 10 minutes Natural, then Quick

Total Time: 20 to 25 minutes

SIMPLE SWAP: If you don't want to use this Mediterranean version of cocktail sauce, try pairing the shrimp with Basil-Walnut Pesto (page 150), or pair with any sauce you like.

PER SERVING: Calories: 130; Fat: 3g; Carbohydrates: 3g; Fiber: 0g; Sugar: 0g; Protein: 23g; Sodium: 235mg

TO MAKE THE SHRIMP

1. Fill a medium bowl with ice water.

2. In the electric pressure cooker, combine the shrimp, water, and salt. Mix well. Secure the lid, and cook on low pressure for 1 minute.

3. After cooking, let the pressure release naturally for 10 minutes, then quick release the remaining pressure. Unlock and remove the lid.

4. Drain the shrimp in a colander, then immediately place in the ice water bath to stop cooking.

TO MAKE THE COCKTAIL SAUCE

5. While the shrimp is cooking, in a small bowl, mix together the water, harissa, mint, and lemon juice.

6. Serve the shrimp with the cocktail sauce on the side.

COLD-POACHED SALMON SALAD

This poached salmon dish is a delicious lunch or light dinner. Salmon characteristics may vary with the species, ranging in color from orange to pink or red. Widely known as an excellent source of brain-boosting omega-3 fatty acids, salmon is also rich in protein, potassium, selenium, and vitamin B_{12}.

1½ cups Vegetable Stock (page 148) or store-bought vegetable stock

½ cup white wine

1 lemon, thinly sliced

1 bay leaf

Olive oil cooking spray, for coating the steam rack

2 (6-ounce) salmon fillets

½ teaspoon kosher salt

¼ teaspoon freshly ground black pepper

1 head Boston or Bibb lettuce

1 cup sliced radishes

1 cup cherry tomatoes, halved

¼ cup Tahini Dressing (page 151)

SERVES 2

DAIRY-FREE, GLUTEN-FREE

Prep Time: 15 minutes

Pressure Cook: 4 minutes

Pressure Level: Low

Release: Quick

Total Time: 30 to 35 minutes, plus 1 hour to chill

SAVE FOR LATER: Salmon can be cooked ahead and kept in the refrigerator up to 24 hours prior to serving.

PER SERVING: Calories: 470; Fat: 32g; Carbohydrates: 7g; Fiber: 3g; Sugar: 3g; Protein: 38g; Sodium: 550mg

1. In the electric pressure cooker, combine the stock, wine, lemon, and bay leaf.

2. Coat a steam rack with cooking spray, and put it inside the pot, handles extending up. Place the salmon fillets, skin-side down, on the prepared steam rack. Season with the salt and pepper.

3. Secure the lid, and cook on low pressure for 4 minutes.

4. After cooking, quick release the pressure. Unlock and remove the lid.

5. Carefully remove the inner pot, and let sit at room temperature for 10 minutes. Then refrigerate for 1 hour.

6. Split the lettuce between 2 large plates.

7. Divide the salmon fillets, radishes, and tomatoes between the plates.

8. Drizzle with the dressing, and serve.

TUNA NIÇOISE SALAD

Tuna Niçoise salad originated in France in the city of Nice. It is often prepared as a composed salad, meaning there is romaine across the bottom, but each remaining ingredient is placed in its own area on top of the greens. Some versions also contain anchovies or Niçoise olives, which would make a delicious addition to this recipe as well.

FOR THE EGGS, POTATOES, AND GREEN BEANS

8 ounces mini potatoes, halved

8 ounces green beans, trimmed

2 large eggs

FOR THE SALAD

1 head romaine lettuce, chopped

1 cup cherry tomatoes, halved

1 (7-ounce) jar oil-packed tuna, drained

¼ cup Tahini Dressing (page 151)

SERVES 2

DAIRY-FREE, GLUTEN-FREE

Prep Time: 20 minutes

Pressure Cook: 3 minutes

Pressure Level: High

Release: Quick

Total Time: 30 to 35 minutes

SIMPLE SWAP: Feel free to use whatever dressing you like. A simple mix of oil and vinegar is always great!

PER SERVING: Calories: 600; Fat: 32g; Carbohydrates: 42g; Fiber: 13g; Sugar: 12g; Protein: 44g; Sodium: 465mg

TO MAKE THE EGGS, POTATOES, AND GREEN BEANS

1. Fill a large bowl with ice water.

2. Pour 1 cup of water into the electric pressure cooker. Place the potatoes, green beans, and eggs in a steamer basket. Gently place in the pot. Secure the lid, and cook on high pressure for 3 minutes.

3. After cooking, quick release the pressure. Unlock and remove the lid.

4. Transfer the vegetables and eggs to the ice water bath.

5. Peel and halve the eggs.

TO MAKE THE SALAD

6. While everything is cooking, arrange the lettuce on a serving platter.

7. Place the tomatoes, eggs, green beans, potatoes, and tuna on top.

8. Serve the salad topped with the dressing.

SALMON WITH BASIL-WALNUT PESTO

These salmon fillets are topped with a tasty basil-walnut pesto sauce, which is an easy and delicious way to get those heart-healthy omega-3 fatty acids! If you prefer to have individual portions prepped prior to cooking, simply cut the salmon fillet into four pieces or purchase four separate 5-ounce portions. Serve with Basic Brown Rice (page 142) or Greek-Style Lentils (page 50).

½ cup Vegetable Stock (page 148) or store-bought vegetable stock

½ cup loosely packed fresh parsley

Olive oil cooking spray, for coating the steam rack

1⅓ pounds salmon fillets, about 1-inch thick

½ teaspoon kosher salt

¼ teaspoon freshly ground black pepper

¼ cup Basil-Walnut Pesto (page 150) or store-bought pesto

SERVES 4

GLUTEN-FREE

Prep Time: 5 minutes

Pressure Cook: 3 minutes

Pressure Level: Low

Release: Quick

Total Time: 10 to 15 minutes

SIMPLE SWAP: Not a fan of salmon or simply looking to try a different variety of fish? Arctic char and cod are both great options.

PER SERVING: Calories: 400; Fat: 29g; Carbohydrates: 1g; Fiber: 0g; Sugar: 0g; Protein: 33g; Sodium: 320mg

1. In the electric pressure cooker, combine the stock and parsley.

2. Coat the steam rack with cooking spray, and put it inside the pot, handles extending up. Place the salmon, skin-side down, on the prepared steam rack. Season with salt and pepper.

3. Secure the lid, and cook on low pressure for 3 minutes.

4. After cooking, quick release the pressure. Unlock and remove the lid.

5. Carefully remove the steam rack with the salmon.

6. Cut the salmon into 4 portions.

7. Top each portion with 1 tablespoon of pesto.

WHOLE BRANZINO

Branzino has been called European bass and is very popular in Mediterranean cuisine. Cooking and serving a whole fish doesn't have to be reserved for restaurant meals! This simple, tasty, and healthy recipe can easily be made any day of the week. To round out the meal, serve it with Braised Fennel (page 38) and Farro with Herby Yogurt (page 48).

1 whole branzino, cleaned and scaled

½ teaspoon kosher salt

¼ teaspoon freshly ground black pepper

Olive oil cooking spray, for coating the steam rack

1 lemon, thinly sliced

SERVES 2

DAIRY-FREE, GLUTEN-FREE

Prep Time: 5 minutes

Pressure Cook: 7 minutes

Pressure Level: High

Release: Quick

Total Time: 20 to 25 minutes

1. Season the inside of the branzino with the salt and pepper.

2. Pour 1 cup of water into the electric pressure cooker.

3. Coat a steam rack with cooking spray, and put it inside the pot, handles extending up. Place the branzino on the prepared steam rack.

4. Place half of the lemon slices on top of the fish.

5. Secure the lid, and cook on high pressure for 7 minutes.

6. After cooking, quick release the pressure. Unlock and remove the lid.

7. Carefully remove the steam rack with the branzino.

8. Place the branzino on a serving platter with the remaining lemon slices. Remove the fillets; they should easily separate and pull away from the bones. Serve immediately.

SIMPLE SWAP: Any whole fish or large side of fish or fillet that can fit in your electric pressure cooker would work well with this recipe. Just be sure the fish you choose has been cleaned and scaled.

PER SERVING: Calories: 220; Fat: 7g; Carbohydrates: 0g; Fiber: 0g; Sugar: 0g; Protein: 36g; Sodium: 365mg

SHRIMP WITH LENTILS

This hearty meal provides a full range of healthy fats, lean protein, and complex carbohydrates—and it's easy to make and tastes delicious. Lentils are an affordable legume, providing dietary fiber and complex carbohydrates as well as vitamins and minerals such as folate and manganese. Shrimp is an excellent source of lean protein, zinc, and magnesium. Rounding out the dish is an assortment of vegetables, providing even more nutrients.

1 tablespoon extra-virgin olive oil

1 onion, diced

1 carrot, diced

1 bell pepper, diced

3 garlic cloves, minced

1 teaspoon kosher salt

1 tablespoon sweet paprika

¼ teaspoon red pepper flakes

1 pound plum tomatoes, chopped

2½ cups Vegetable Stock (page 148) or store-bought vegetable stock

1 cup dried French green lentils

1 pound shrimp, peeled and deveined

Juice of 1 lemon

1 tablespoon tahini (optional)

SERVES 4

DAIRY-FREE, GLUTEN-FREE

Prep Time: 20 minutes

Pressure Cook: 20 minutes

Pressure Level: High

Release: 10 minutes Natural, then Quick

Total Time: 1 hour 10 minutes

SIMPLE SWAP: Feel free to swap out the plum tomatoes for 1 (14½-ounce) can diced tomatoes. The stock can also be replaced with water.

PER SERVING: Calories: 365; Fat: 7g; Carbohydrates: 43g; Fiber: 11g; Sugar: 9g; Protein: 35g; Sodium: 555mg

1. Press the sauté button on the electric pressure cooker, allow it to heat up, then add the oil.

2. Add the onion, carrot, and bell pepper. Sauté for 3 minutes, or until softened.

3. Add the garlic, salt, paprika, and red pepper flakes. Sauté for 30 seconds, or until fragrant.

4. Add the tomatoes, stock, and lentils. Mix well. Press the cancel button to stop cooking.

5. Secure the lid, and cook on high pressure for 20 minutes.

6. After cooking, let the pressure release naturally for 10 minutes, then quick release the remaining pressure. Unlock and remove the lid, then mix well.

7. Add the shrimp, and place the lid askew over the pot. Press the sauté button, and simmer for about 4 minutes, or until the shrimp has cooked through. Press the cancel button to stop cooking.

8. Add the lemon juice, and mix well.

9. Serve the shrimp and lentils drizzled with the tahini (if using).

HALIBUT WITH TOMATO-CHILE SAUCE

The fiery tomato-chile sauce in this dish pairs well with a hearty white fish like halibut; the added touch of rich tahini at the end helps counter some of the heat. The sauce can be batched up and saved for a future use. Simply remove half after step 7, put in an airtight container, and freeze for up to 6 months. It will also taste scrumptious on top of roasted poultry or mixed in with whole grains.

2 tablespoons extra-virgin olive oil

1 jalapeño or red chile, seeded and finely diced

4 garlic cloves, sliced

1½ pounds plum tomatoes, diced

1 poblano pepper, seeded and diced

3 tablespoons tomato paste

1 teaspoon kosher salt

1 teaspoon ground cumin

½ teaspoon honey

½ cup water, Vegetable Stock (page 148), or store-bought vegetable stock

4 (6-ounce) halibut fillets

¼ cup chopped fresh cilantro

2 tablespoons tahini

SERVES 4

DAIRY-FREE, GLUTEN-FREE

Prep Time: 15 minutes

Pressure Cook: 2 minutes

Pressure Level: High

Release: Quick

Total Time: 40 to 45 minutes

SIMPLE SWAP: This recipe works well with any hearty white fish. Feel free to swap out the halibut for whatever you prefer, such as cod or bass.

PER SERVING: Calories: 340; Fat: 15g; Carbohydrates: 13g; Fiber: 4g; Sugar: 8g; Protein: 39g; Sodium: 420mg

1. Press the sauté button on the electric pressure cooker, allow it to heat up, then add the oil.

2. Add the jalapeño, and sauté for 1 minute.

3. Add the garlic, and sauté for 30 seconds, or until fragrant.

4. Add the tomatoes and poblano pepper. Cook for 3 minutes, or until softened.

5. Add the tomato paste, salt, cumin, and honey. Sauté for 1 minute.

6. Add the water, and deglaze: mix well, and scrape up any brown bits on the bottom of the pot. Press the cancel button to stop cooking.

7. Secure the lid, and cook on high pressure for 2 minutes.

8. After cooking, quick release the pressure. Unlock and remove the lid, then mix well.

9. Nestle the halibut fillets into the mixture. Press the sauté button, place the lid askew over the pot, and simmer for 10 to 12 minutes, or until the halibut is cooked through and opaque. Press the cancel button to stop cooking.

10. Serve the halibut garnished with the cilantro and drizzled with the tahini.

MONKFISH WITH KALE AND WHITE BEANS

Monkfish has often been called the "poor man's lobster" and can be found across the Mediterranean Sea, particularly along the coast of Europe. It has a mild, slightly sweet taste and is dense, firm, and boneless, similar to lobster tail. Its firm texture means that it will not fall apart when cooked, so it typically holds up very well in the electric pressure cooker.

2 tablespoons extra-virgin olive oil

1 onion, diced

1 tablespoon minced fresh rosemary leaves

2 garlic cloves, minced

¾ teaspoon kosher salt

¼ teaspoon red pepper flakes

1 bunch kale, stemmed and chopped

2 cups Basic Beans (page 143) or canned cannellini beans

½ cup white wine

½ cup Vegetable Stock (page 148) or store-bought vegetable stock

1 pound monkfish

Juice of ½ lemon

SERVES 4

DAIRY-FREE, GLUTEN-FREE

Prep Time: 15 minutes
Pressure Cook: 5 minutes
Pressure Level: High
Release: 10 minutes Natural, then Quick
Total Time: 45 minutes

HELPFUL HACK: Pre-packaged chopped kale or baby kale can be used in place of the regular bunch of kale, which may cut down on prep time. Other greens, such as Swiss chard or spinach, may be used in place of the kale as well.

PER SERVING: Calories: 330; Fat: 9g; Carbohydrates: 30g; Fiber: 8g; Sugar: 3g; Protein: 27g; Sodium: 270mg

1. Press the sauté button on the electric pressure cooker, allow it to heat up, then add the oil.

2. Add the onion, and sauté for 2 minutes, or until softened.

3. Add the rosemary, garlic, salt, and red pepper flakes. Sauté for 30 seconds, or until fragrant.

4. Add the kale, and sauté for 2 minutes, or until wilted.

5. Add the beans, and sauté for 1 minute.

6. Add the wine, and deglaze: mix well, and scrape up any brown bits on the bottom of the pot.

7. Add the stock, and mix well.

8. Nestle the monkfish in the pot. Press the cancel button to stop cooking.

9. Secure the lid, and cook on high pressure for 5 minutes.

10. After cooking, let the pressure release naturally for 10 minutes, then quick release the remaining pressure. Unlock and remove the lid, then mix well. The fish should be cooked through and opaque. If it is not quite cooked through, press the sauté button, place the lid askew over pot, and simmer until finished. Press the cancel button to stop cooking.

11. Add the lemon juice, and mix well. Serve.

COD WITH PUTTANESCA

Puttanesca is an Italian sauce composed of capers and olives. It is typically tossed with pasta; however, it pairs beautifully with hearty white fish like cod. I've added some anchovy paste for an extra briny kick, but you can remove that completely or replace it with some chopped jarred anchovies. The heat can be eased up or kicked up a notch by adjusting the amount of red pepper flakes.

1 tablespoon extra-virgin olive oil

3 garlic cloves, minced

1 tablespoon tomato paste

1 teaspoon anchovy paste

½ teaspoon kosher salt

¼ teaspoon red pepper flakes

1 (28-ounce) can low-sodium whole tomatoes, crushed with hands

½ cup water

⅓ cup chopped fresh basil leaves

⅓ cup chopped pitted Kalamata olives

1 tablespoon capers, drained and rinsed

4 (6-ounce) cod fillets

¼ cup chopped fresh parsley

SERVES 4

DAIRY-FREE, GLUTEN-FREE

Prep Time: 15 minutes

Pressure Cook: 3 minutes

Pressure Level: High

Release: Quick

Total Time: 35 to 40 minutes

SIMPLE SWAP: Any type of fish fillets you like should work well in place of the cod fillets.

PER SERVING: Calories: 225; Fat: 6g; Carbohydrates: 10g; Fiber: 2g; Sugar: 5g; Protein: 32g; Sodium: 540mg

1. Press the sauté function on the electric pressure cooker, allow it to heat up, then add the oil.

2. Add the garlic, and sauté for 30 seconds, or until fragrant.

3. Add the tomato paste, anchovy paste, salt, and red pepper flakes. Sauté for 30 seconds.

4. Add the tomatoes with their juices, water, basil, olives, and capers. Mix well. Press the cancel button to stop cooking.

5. Secure the lid, and cook on high pressure for 3 minutes.

6. After cooking, quick release the pressure. Unlock and remove the lid, then mix well.

7. Add the cod fillets, and place the lid askew over the pot. Press the sauté button, and simmer for about 10 minutes, or until the cod is cooked through and opaque. Press the cancel button to stop cooking.

8. Garnish with the parsley, and serve.

CHAPTER SEVEN

POULTRY AND MEAT

OSSO BUCO Page 106

SAUSAGE-BEAN SOUP

Browning the sausage adds a flavorful depth to the finished dish. Cooking the sausage whole before slicing helps it keep its texture intact, a welcome addition to this delicious soup. To ramp up the vegetables, mix in some chopped spinach or Swiss chard at the end with the lemon juice.

2 tablespoons vegetable oil, divided

1 pound hot or sweet sausage

1 onion, diced

1 carrot, diced

1 celery stalk, diced

2 garlic cloves, minced

¾ teaspoon kosher salt

½ teaspoon dried thyme

½ teaspoon dried sage

¼ teaspoon freshly ground black pepper

4 cups Chicken Stock (page 149) or store-bought gluten-free chicken stock

1½ cups dried kidney beans

1 bay leaf

Juice of 1 lemon

Pita or crusty bread, for serving

SERVES 6
DAIRY-FREE, GLUTEN-FREE

Prep Time: 20 minutes
Pressure Cook: 30 minutes
Pressure Level: High
Release: 20 minutes Natural, then Quick
Total Time: 1 hour 30 minutes

SIMPLE SWAP: Any beans you like will taste great in this soup. Just swap out the kidney beans, and add a different dried bean.

PER SERVING: Calories: 330; Fat: 11g; Carbohydrates: 34g; Fiber: 12g; Sugar: 3g; Protein: 25g; Sodium: 990mg

1. Press the sauté button on the electric pressure cooker, allow it to heat up, then add 1 tablespoon of oil.

2. Add the sausage, and cook, turning, for about 3 minutes, or until brown on all sides. Transfer to a cutting board. Cut into bite-size rounds.

3. Add the remaining 1 tablespoon of oil, the onion, carrot, and celery to the pot. Sauté for 3 minutes, or until the vegetables start to soften.

4. Add the garlic, salt, thyme, sage, and pepper. Sauté for 30 seconds, or until fragrant.

5. Add the stock, beans, bay leaf, and sausage. Press the cancel button to stop cooking.

6. Secure the lid, and cook on high pressure for 30 minutes.

7. After cooking, let the pressure release naturally for 20 minutes, then quick release the remaining pressure. Unlock and remove the lid.

8. Add lemon juice. Mix well.

9. Serve the soup warm with some pita or crusty bread.

GREEN CHICKEN SOUP

Chicken soup gets an upgrade with the addition of some delicious, nutritious, and beautiful green vegetables. This dish is perfect for spring, when all the fresh green produce appears at the farmers' market. To make it heartier, mix in some Basic Brown Rice (page 142) or Basic Beans (page 143).

2 pounds bone-in chicken thighs, skin removed

4 cups Chicken Stock (page 149) or store-bought gluten-free chicken stock

1 pound asparagus, woody ends trimmed, cut into ½-inch pieces

10 ounces frozen peas

1 onion, diced

2 celery stalks, diced

1 teaspoon dried thyme

¾ teaspoon kosher salt

¼ teaspoon freshly ground black pepper

1 bay leaf

1 bunch Swiss chard, stemmed and chopped

Crusty bread, for serving (optional)

SERVES 6

DAIRY-FREE, GLUTEN-FREE

Prep Time: 20 minutes

Pressure Cook: 20 minutes

Pressure Level: High

Release: 20 minutes Natural, then Quick

Total Time: 1 hour 10 minutes

SIMPLE SWAP: If fresh peas are available, they make a great addition in place of the frozen peas.

PER SERVING: Calories: 250; Fat: 7g; Carbohydrates: 11g; Fiber: 3g; Sugar: 5g; Protein: 34g; Sodium: 780mg

1. In the electric pressure cooker, combine the chicken, stock, asparagus, peas, onion, celery, thyme, salt, pepper, and bay leaf. Mix well. Secure the lid, and cook on high pressure for 20 minutes.

2. After cooking, let the pressure release naturally for 20 minutes, then quick release the remaining pressure. Unlock and remove the lid.

3. Transfer the chicken to a cutting board. Take the meat off the bone, and return the meat to the pot.

4. Add the Swiss chard, and mix well.

5. Ladle the soup into bowls. Serve with crusty bread, if desired.

AVGOLEMONO (GREEK CHICKEN AND EGG SOUP)

Avgolemono is basically a Greek version of chicken and rice soup that is thickened with egg yolks. It is a bright, light dish that is perfect for a lunch or low-key dinner. Drizzle with extra-virgin olive oil before serving.

4 cups Chicken Stock (page 149) or store-bought gluten-free chicken stock

1 pound boneless, skinless chicken breasts

¾ teaspoon kosher salt

½ teaspoon dried thyme

½ teaspoon dried oregano

¼ teaspoon freshly ground black pepper

2 cups Basic Brown Rice (page 142), divided

3 tablespoons freshly squeezed lemon juice

2 large egg yolks

2 tablespoons chopped fresh dill

SERVES 6

DAIRY-FREE, GLUTEN-FREE

Prep Time: 15 minutes

Pressure Cook: 15 minutes

Pressure Level: High

Release: Quick

Total Time: 40 to 45 minutes

TROUBLESHOOTING TIP: The egg yolk mixture is meant to help thicken the soup. If the soup does not thicken after 5 minutes of simmering in step 7, continue to simmer another 5 minutes, and stir occasionally.

PER SERVING: Calories: 190; Fat: 4g; Carbohydrates: 16g; Fiber: 1g; Sugar: 1g; Protein: 21g; Sodium: 580mg

1. In the electric pressure cooker, combine the stock, chicken, salt, thyme, oregano, and pepper. Mix well. Secure the lid, and cook on high pressure for 15 minutes.

2. After cooking, quick release the pressure. Unlock and remove the lid.

3. Transfer the chicken to a cutting board. Shred using 2 forks.

4. In a blender, process ½ cup of rice, the lemon juice, and egg yolks.

5. Slowly add 1 cup of the hot broth from the electric pressure cooker, and continue to process.

6. Add the mixture to the electric pressure cooker along with the shredded chicken and remaining 1½ cups of brown rice.

7. Press the sauté button, and simmer for 5 minutes, or until the soup has thickened. Press the cancel button to stop cooking.

8. Garnish the soup with dill before serving.

OSSO BUCO

Osso buco is a classic braised veal dish from northern Italy whose name literally translates to "bone with a hole." The cut of veal used has a round, marrow-filled bone that is a special treat. Be sure to grab a small spoon to try that silky bone marrow on a piece of crusty bread. This delicious, hearty meal tastes amazing when it's made and even better the next day! Pair it with Basic Brown Rice (page 142) to round out the meal and garnish with fresh herbs if desired.

2 to 2½ pounds osso buco (4 pieces)

1 teaspoon kosher salt

½ teaspoon freshly ground black pepper

½ cup all-purpose flour

3 tablespoons extra-virgin olive oil, divided

3 carrots, diced

1 onion, diced

2 celery stalks, diced

5 garlic cloves, sliced

1 tablespoon tomato paste

½ cup red wine

1 (28-ounce) can low-sodium whole tomatoes

½ cup beef stock

4 thyme sprigs

2 rosemary sprigs

1 oregano sprig

1 bay leaf

SERVES 4

DAIRY-FREE

Prep Time: 15 minutes

Pressure Cook: 40 minutes

Pressure Level: High

Release: 20 minutes Natural, then Quick

Total Time: 2 hours 5 minutes

SIMPLE SWAP: Dried herbs can be used in place of the fresh: simply use ¼ teaspoon oregano, ½ teaspoon thyme, and ½ teaspoon rosemary.

PER SERVING: Calories: 490; Fat: 17g; Carbohydrates: 31g; Fiber: 5g; Sugar: 10g; Protein: 49g; Sodium: 600mg

1. Season the osso buco all over with the salt and pepper.

2. Dredge the osso buco in the flour.

3. Press the sauté button on the electric pressure cooker, allow it to heat up, then add 2 tablespoons of oil.

4. Add the osso buco, and cook for about 5 minutes per side, or until browned all over. Remove the osso buco, and set aside.

5. In the electric pressure cooker, combine the carrots, onion, celery, and remaining 1 tablespoon of oil. Sauté for 8 minutes, or until softened.

6. Add the garlic and tomato paste. Sauté for 30 seconds, or until fragrant.

7. Add the wine, and deglaze: mix well, and scrape up any brown bits on the bottom of the pot.

8. Add the tomatoes with their juices, stock, thyme, rosemary, oregano, and bay leaf. Mix well.

9. Nestle the osso buco into the mixture. Press the cancel button to stop cooking.

10. Secure the lid, and cook on high pressure for 40 minutes.

11. After cooking, let the pressure release naturally for 20 minutes, then quick release the remaining pressure. Unlock and remove the lid.

12. Carefully remove the herb sprigs and osso buco, and set aside.

13. Press the sauté button, and simmer the sauce for at least 10 minutes, or until reduced to your desired consistency. Press the cancel button to stop cooking.

14. Return the osso buco to the pot, and serve.

MEDITERRANEAN-STYLE BRISKET

Brisket is a cut of beef that is found just below the shoulder, making it more muscular and a tougher cut. Pressure cooking with moist heat transforms the brisket into a tender, juicy cut of meat. When cooked, the brisket can be cut into uniform pieces or pulled apart in a more shredded fashion. Any way you slice it, the result will be amazingly delicious!

6 garlic cloves, minced

1 teaspoon dried oregano

1 teaspoon kosher salt

½ teaspoon red pepper flakes

½ teaspoon freshly ground black pepper

1 (2- to 3-pound) beef brisket

1 tablespoon grapeseed oil

3 carrots, cut into ½-inch pieces

2 parsnips, cut into ½-inch pieces

1 onion, julienned

2 celery stalks, cut into ½-inch pieces

¼ cup red-wine vinegar

1 (14½-ounce) can low-sodium diced tomatoes

1½ cups gluten-free beef broth

1 strip orange zest

1 cinnamon stick

½ cup chopped fresh parsley

SERVES 8

DAIRY-FREE, GLUTEN-FREE

Prep Time: 1 hour

Pressure Cook: 1 hour 15 minutes

Pressure Level: High

Release: 30 minutes Natural, then Quick

Total Time: 3 hours 15 minutes

SIMPLE SWAP: A variety of root vegetables will work well in this dish. Feel free to swap out the carrots or parsnips for turnips and sweet potatoes.

PER SERVING: Calories: 465; Fat: 33g; Carbohydrates: 11g; Fiber: 3g; Sugar: 5g; Protein: 27g; Sodium: 360mg

1. In a small bowl, mix together the garlic, oregano, salt, red pepper flakes, and pepper.

2. Season the brisket all over with the mixture. Let sit at room temperature for 1 hour.

3. Press the sauté button on the electric pressure cooker, allow it to heat up, then add the oil.

4. Add the brisket, and cook for about 5 minutes on one side, or until browned. Remove the brisket, and set aside.

5. Add the carrots, parsnips, onion, and celery. Sauté for 3 minutes, or until softened.

6. Add the vinegar, and deglaze: mix well, and scrape up any brown bits on the bottom of the pot.

7. Add the tomatoes with their juices, broth, zest, and cinnamon. Mix well.

8. Nestle the brisket into the mixture. Press the cancel button to stop cooking.

9. Secure the lid, and cook on high pressure for 1 hour 15 minutes.

10. After cooking, let the pressure release naturally for 30 minutes, then quick release the remaining pressure. Unlock and remove the lid.

11. Transfer the brisket to a cutting board.

12. Press the sauté button, and simmer the sauce for at least 10 minutes, or until reduced to your desired consistency. Press the cancel button to stop cooking.

13. Slice the brisket, and serve with the sauce and vegetables.

14. Garnish with the parsley.

MOROCCAN LAMB

Ras el hanout is a Moroccan spice blend whose name translates to "head of the shop." This aromatic, flavorful spice blend typically contains cinnamon, cumin, coriander, allspice, black pepper, ginger, and salt. Look for it in the spice aisle of your grocery store or find it online. It pairs beautifully with the lamb, and the apricots and pomegranate provide a bright, sweet pop of flavor to round out the dish.

2 tablespoons ras el hanout, divided

¾ teaspoon kosher salt

1 pound lamb shanks

1 tablespoon extra-virgin olive oil

1 onion, julienned

5 garlic cloves, minced

1½ cups gluten-free beef broth

2 cups Basic Chickpeas (page 143) or canned chickpeas

½ cup chopped dried apricots

½ cup chopped fresh cilantro

½ cup pomegranate seeds

SERVES 4

DAIRY-FREE, GLUTEN-FREE

Prep Time: 15 minutes

Pressure Cook: 45 minutes

Pressure Level: High

Release: 20 minutes Natural, then Quick

Total Time: 1 hour 40 minutes

SAVE FOR LATER: Once you are done eating, save the lamb shank bones and make lamb stock. Just look at the recipe for Chicken Stock (page 149) and swap out the chicken bones for lamb bones.

PER SERVING: Calories: 385; Fat: 9g; Carbohydrates: 45g; Fiber: 9g; Sugar: 20g; Protein: 32g; Sodium: 550mg

1. In a small bowl, mix together 1 tablespoon of ras el hanout and the salt.

2. Season the lamb shanks all over with the mixture.

3. Press the sauté button on the electric pressure cooker, allow it to heat up, then add the oil.

4. Add the onion, and sauté for 3 minutes, or until softened.

5. Add the garlic and remaining 1 tablespoon of ras el hanout. Sauté for 30 seconds, or until fragrant.

6. Add the broth, and deglaze: mix well, and scrape up any brown bits on the bottom of the pot.

7. Nestle the lamb shanks into the mixture. Press the cancel button to stop cooking.

8. Secure the lid, and cook on high pressure for 45 minutes.

9. After cooking, let the pressure release naturally for 20 minutes, then quick release the remaining pressure. Unlock and remove the lid.

10. Transfer the lamb to a cutting board. Remove the meat from the bone, reserving the bone (see tip).

11. Stir in the chickpeas and dried apricots. Press the sauté button, and simmer the sauce for about 5 minutes, or until thickened.

12. Add the lamb meat to the electric pressure cooker. Press the cancel button to stop cooking.

13. Serve the lamb garnished with the cilantro and pomegranate seeds.

WHOLE CHICKEN

There's something cozy about a juicy, tender whole chicken. My recipe takes some hands-on time, but it's worth it! Sautéing helps lock in the flavor and gives it a golden brown hue, making it look even more appetizing. Feel free to swap out the herbs for whatever you like and have on hand. Serve with Potatoes with Greens (page 41) or Farro with Herby Yogurt (page 48).

1 (3- to 4-pound) whole chicken, giblets removed

2 teaspoons kosher salt

1 teaspoon freshly ground black pepper

1 tablespoon extra-virgin olive oil

½ cup water

6 garlic cloves, peeled

1 bunch rosemary, thyme, or sage

SERVES 6

DAIRY-FREE, GLUTEN-FREE

Prep Time: 5 minutes

Pressure Cook: 30 minutes

Pressure Level: High

Release: 15 minutes Natural, then Quick

Total Time: 1 hour 20 minutes

1. Season the chicken with the salt and pepper.

2. Press the sauté button on the electric pressure cooker, allow it to heat up, then add the oil.

3. Add the chicken, breast-side down, and cook for 5 minutes. Do not move the chicken!

4. Using tongs or 2 large spoons, carefully turn it over, and cook for another 5 minutes, or until browned. Press the cancel button to stop cooking.

5. Add the water, carefully drop in the garlic, and lay the rosemary around and across the top of the chicken.

6. Secure the lid, and cook on high pressure for 30 minutes.

7. After cooking, let the pressure release naturally for 15 minutes, then quick release the remaining pressure. Unlock and remove the lid.

8. Transfer the chicken to a large cutting board. Let rest for another 10 minutes, then cut and serve.

SAVE FOR LATER: Leftover chicken has countless possibilities! Add it to soup, stew, salads, and more; it will keep in the refrigerator for 5 days. Once all the meat has been cut off the chicken carcass, put the carcass in a resealable freezer bag, label and date the bag, and freeze for up to 3 months. Once you are ready, use the leftover chicken bones to make Chicken Stock (page 149).

PER SERVING: Calories: 255; Fat: 25g; Carbohydrates: 1g; Fiber: 0g; Sugar: 0g; Protein: 29g; Sodium: 480mg

SHREDDED CHICKEN WITH HARISSA

Harissa is a flavorful, aromatic chili pepper paste or sauce that is widely used in some Mediterranean regions, specifically North African and Middle Eastern countries. This recipe can be mild, medium, or spicy depending on the harissa you choose. Pair with Tzatziki (page 147) for a refreshing combination that is sure to delight.

1 pound boneless, skinless chicken breasts

1 cup Chicken Stock (page 149) or store-bought gluten-free chicken stock

⅓ cup harissa

½ teaspoon kosher salt

¼ teaspoon freshly ground black pepper

1. In the electric pressure cooker, combine the chicken, stock, harissa, salt, and pepper. Mix well. Secure the lid, and cook on high pressure for 25 minutes.

2. After cooking, let the pressure release naturally for 20 minutes, then quick release the remaining pressure. Unlock and remove the lid.

3. Using 2 forks, shred the chicken. Serve immediately.

SERVES 4

DAIRY-FREE, GLUTEN-FREE

Prep Time: 10 minutes

Pressure Cook: 25 minutes

Pressure Level: High

Release: 20 minutes Natural, then Quick

Total Time: 1 hour 5 minutes

SIMPLE SWAP: Boneless, skinless chicken thighs can be used in place of the chicken breasts.

PER SERVING: Calories: 150; Fat: 4g; Carbohydrates: 2g; Fiber: 0g; Sugar: 0g; Protein: 26g; Sodium: 425mg

LAMB MEATLOAF WITH TAHINI SAUCE

A mini loaf pan fits this lamb meatloaf perfectly in an electric pressure cooker. If you don't have a mini loaf pan, a 7-inch round cake pan works well. Pair this scrumptious recipe with Potatoes with Greens (page 41) for a well-balanced Mediterranean meal.

Olive oil cooking spray, for coating the loaf pan

1 pound ground lamb

⅓ cup bread crumbs

¼ cup Vegetable Stock (page 148) or store-bought vegetable stock

¼ cup minced onion

¼ cup minced fresh mint leaves

1 large egg, beaten

1 garlic clove, minced

2 teaspoons ground cumin

1 teaspoon ground coriander

1 teaspoon kosher salt, divided

½ teaspoon freshly ground black pepper

½ teaspoon ground cinnamon

½ cup Plain Yogurt (page 145) or store-bought plain yogurt

⅓ cup tahini

¼ cup freshly squeezed lemon juice

SERVES 4

Prep Time: 15 minutes
Pressure Cook: 25 minutes
Pressure Level: High
Release: 20 minutes Natural, then Quick
Total Time: 1 hour 20 minutes

TROUBLESHOOTING TIP:
To ensure lamb is cooked through properly, use an instant-read thermometer. It should register at least 160°F.

PER SERVING: Calories: 535; Fat: 38g; Carbohydrates: 19g; Fiber: 3g; Sugar: 5g; Protein: 28g; Sodium: 435mg

1. Spray a mini loaf pan with cooking spray.

2. In a medium bowl, mix together the lamb, bread crumbs, stock, onion, mint, egg, garlic, cumin, coriander, ½ teaspoon of salt, pepper, and cinnamon.

3. Pack the mixture into the prepared loaf pan, and cover tightly with aluminum foil.

4. Pour 1½ cups of water into the electric pressure cooker, place the steam trivet inside, and place the loaf pan on top of the trivet. Secure the lid, and cook on high pressure for 25 minutes.

5. After cooking, let the pressure release naturally for 20 minutes, then quick release the remaining pressure. Unlock and remove the lid. Remove the loaf pan, uncover, and let cool for 10 minutes.

6. While the lamb is cooking, to make the tahini sauce, in a small bowl, mix together the yogurt, tahini, lemon juice, and remaining ½ teaspoon of salt.

7. Pour the tahini sauce over the meatloaf, or serve on the side.

CHICKEN WITH MUSHROOMS

Mushrooms add an earthy flavor to this dish, pair beautifully with chicken, and are an excellent source of many nutrients, including selenium, zinc, B vitamins, and potassium. Serve with lemon wedges and a sprinkle of parsley for an extra pop.

4 bone-in chicken breasts, skin removed (2 to 2½ pounds)

1 teaspoon kosher salt

¼ teaspoon freshly ground black pepper

2 tablespoons extra-virgin olive oil, divided

1 pound cremini mushrooms, thinly sliced

1 onion, diced

1 cup Chicken Stock (page 149) or store-bought gluten-free chicken stock

1 tablespoon Italian seasoning

SERVES 4

DAIRY-FREE, GLUTEN-FREE

Prep Time: 15 minutes

Pressure Cook: 15 minutes

Pressure Level: High

Release: Quick

Total Time: 50 to 55 minutes

SIMPLE SWAP: Feel free to swap out the chicken breasts for bone-in, skinless chicken thighs and drumsticks.

PER SERVING: Calories: 375; Fat: 13g; Carbohydrates: 9g; Fiber: 1g; Sugar: 4g; Protein: 55g; Sodium: 540mg

1. Season the chicken with the salt and pepper.

2. Press the sauté button on the electric pressure cooker, allow it to heat up, then add 1 tablespoon of oil.

3. Add the chicken, and cook on one side for about 5 minutes, or until browned. Remove the chicken, and set aside.

4. Heat the remaining 1 tablespoon of oil.

5. Add the mushrooms and onion. Sauté for 8 to 10 minutes, or until softened.

6. Add the stock and Italian seasoning. Deglaze: mix well, and scrape up any brown bits on the bottom of the pot.

7. Return the chicken to the pressure cooker. Press the cancel button to stop cooking.

8. Secure the lid, and cook on high pressure for 15 minutes.

9. After cooking, quick release the pressure. Unlock and remove the lid.

10. Transfer the chicken to a serving dish. (Optional: Press the sauté button, and simmer the sauce until the desired consistency is reached.) Serve immediately.

LEMON CHICKEN WITH ROSEMARY

Lemon and rosemary are a winning combination in this bright, delicious recipe. Add this dish to Basic Brown Rice (page 142) to soak up the sauce, or pair with Bean Salad (page 46) and some pita bread for a light lunch or dinner. Leftovers can be stored in an airtight container for up to 5 days in the refrigerator or up to 3 months in the freezer.

4 boneless, skinless chicken thighs (1 to 1½ pounds)

1 tablespoon chopped fresh rosemary leaves

1 tablespoon chopped fresh thyme leaves

1 teaspoon kosher salt

¼ teaspoon freshly ground black pepper

1 tablespoon extra-virgin olive oil

½ cup white wine

½ cup Chicken Stock (page 149) or store-bought gluten-free chicken stock

¼ cup freshly squeezed lemon juice

SERVES 4

DAIRY-FREE, GLUTEN-FREE

Prep Time: 10 minutes

Pressure Cook: 15 minutes

Pressure Level: High

Release: Quick

Total Time: 40 to 45 minutes

SIMPLE SWAP: Boneless, skinless chicken breasts can be used in place of the chicken thighs.

PER SERVING: Calories: 260; Fat: 10g; Carbohydrates: 2g; Fiber: 0g; Sugar: 1g; Protein: 34g; Sodium: 515mg

1. Season the chicken with the rosemary, thyme, salt, and pepper.

2. Press the sauté button on the electric pressure cooker, allow it to heat up, then add the oil.

3. Add the chicken, and cook for about 3 minutes per side, or until browned on both sides.

4. Add the wine, stock, and lemon juice. Press the cancel button to stop cooking.

5. Secure the lid, and cook on high pressure for 15 minutes.

6. After cooking, quick release the pressure. Unlock and remove the lid.

7. Using 2 forks, shred the chicken. Serve immediately.

CHICKEN WITH PEPPERS

Bell peppers, available in a range of colors, are widely used throughout the Mediterranean region. Red, orange, and yellow bell peppers are sweeter, whereas green and purple bell peppers have a slightly bitter flavor. Here's a fun fact: Did you know that green bell peppers that are left on the vine to sweeten become red bell peppers? Both paprika and pimento are also prepared from bell peppers.

1 pound boneless, skinless chicken thighs

1 teaspoon kosher salt

¼ teaspoon freshly ground black pepper

2 tablespoons extra-virgin olive oil, divided

1 onion, julienned

1 green bell pepper, julienned

1 red bell pepper, julienned

1 tablespoon fresh oregano leaves or 1 teaspoon dried oregano

2 garlic cloves, minced

½ cup red wine

½ cup Chicken Stock (page 149) or store-bought gluten-free chicken stock

¼ cup chopped fresh parsley

SERVES 4

DAIRY-FREE, GLUTEN-FREE

Prep Time: 20 minutes

Pressure Cook: 15 minutes

Pressure Level: High

Release: Quick

Total Time: 55 minutes to 1 hour

SIMPLE SWAP: Feel free to use any color of bell peppers you like.

PER SERVING: Calories: 255; Fat: 12g; Carbohydrates: 9g; Fiber: 2g; Sugar: 4g; Protein: 24g; Sodium: 465mg

1. Season the chicken with the salt and pepper.

2. Press the sauté button on the electric pressure cooker, allow it to heat up, then add 1 tablespoon of oil.

3. Add the chicken, and cook for 2 to 3 minutes per side, or until browned on both sides. Remove the chicken, and set aside.

4. Heat the remaining 1 tablespoon of oil.

5. Add the onion, green bell pepper, and red bell pepper. Sauté for 5 minutes, or until softened.

6. Add the oregano and garlic. Sauté for 30 seconds, or until fragrant.

7. Add the wine, and deglaze: mix well, and scrape up any brown bits on the bottom of the pot.

8. Add the stock and chicken. Press the cancel button to stop cooking.

9. Secure the lid, and cook on high pressure for 15 minutes.

10. After cooking, quick release the pressure. Unlock and remove the lid.

11. Transfer the chicken to a serving dish. (Optional: Press the sauté button, and simmer the sauce until the desired consistency is reached.)

12. Garnish with the parsley. Serve immediately.

BRAISED CHICKEN WITH TOMATO AND OLIVES

Olives, known as a rich source of healthy fats, are a staple in the Mediterranean diet. They are often cured or pickled by being immersed in water, oil, or brine. Olive oil is made by crushing and pressing olives. Both olives and olive oil are excellent sources of healthy monounsaturated fatty acids, vitamin E, and flavonoids. Garnish the finished dish with parsley, if desired.

4 bone-in chicken thighs, skin removed (2 to 2½ pounds)

1 teaspoon kosher salt

¼ teaspoon freshly ground black pepper

2 tablespoons extra-virgin olive oil, divided

1 onion, diced

1 celery stalk, diced

1 carrot, diced

2 garlic cloves, minced

½ cup white wine

1 (28-ounce) can low-sodium whole tomatoes

¾ cup chopped pitted black olives

¼ cup Chicken Stock (page 149) or store-bought gluten-free chicken stock

2 teaspoons dried basil

2 teaspoons dried oregano

⅛ teaspoon red pepper flakes

SERVES 4
DAIRY-FREE, GLUTEN-FREE

Prep Time: 15 minutes
Pressure Cook: 20 minutes
Pressure Level: High
Release: Quick
Total Time: 55 minutes to 1 hour

SAVE FOR LATER: Leftovers can be stored in an airtight container for up to 5 days in the refrigerator or up to 3 months in the freezer.

PER SERVING: Calories: 450; Fat: 20g; Carbohydrates: 15g; Fiber: 3g; Sugar: 8g; Protein: 47g; Sodium: 900mg

1. Season the chicken with the salt and pepper.

2. Press the sauté button on the electric pressure cooker, allow it to heat up, then add 1 tablespoon of oil.

3. Add the chicken, and cook on one side for about 5 minutes, or until browned. Remove the chicken, and set aside.

4. Heat the remaining 1 tablespoon of oil.

5. Add the onion, celery, and carrot. Sauté for 5 minutes, or until softened.

6. Add the garlic, and sauté for 30 seconds, or until fragrant.

7. Add the wine, and deglaze: mix well, and scrape up any brown bits on the bottom of the pot.

8. Add the tomatoes with their juices, olives, stock, basil, oregano, and red pepper flakes. Mix well.

9. Return the chicken to the pot. Press the cancel button to stop cooking.

10. Secure the lid, and cook on high pressure for 20 minutes.

11. After cooking, quick release the pressure. Unlock and remove the lid.

12. Transfer the chicken to a serving dish. (Optional: Press the sauté button, and simmer the sauce until the desired consistency is reached.) Serve immediately.

MEATBALLS WITH TOMATO SAUCE

The key to making meatballs with the electric pressure cooker is in the bread crumbs. They allow the meatballs to retain a nice texture without getting mushy or falling apart during pressure cooking. Serve the meatballs and tomato sauce over pasta or vegetable noodles, such as zucchini or carrot.

FOR THE MEATBALLS

1 pound ground beef

⅓ cup bread crumbs

⅓ cup grated Parmesan cheese

¼ cup reduced fat milk

1 large egg, beaten

2 tablespoons minced fresh parsley

¾ teaspoon kosher salt

¼ teaspoon freshly ground black pepper

FOR THE SAUCE

1 tablespoon extra-virgin olive oil

1 onion, diced

1 carrot, diced

1 celery stalk, diced

1 tablespoon chopped fresh oregano leaves or 1 teaspoon dried oregano

1 tablespoon chopped fresh basil leaves or 1 teaspoon dried basil

5 garlic cloves, minced

¾ teaspoon kosher salt

¼ teaspoon freshly ground black pepper

2 (28-ounce) cans low-sodium crushed tomatoes

1 teaspoon honey

SERVES 6

Prep Time: 20 minutes

Pressure Cook: 5 minutes

Pressure Level: High

Release: Quick

Total Time: 45 to 55 minutes

SAVE FOR LATER: The meatballs and tomato sauce can be stored in an airtight container for up to 5 days in the refrigerator or up to 3 months in the freezer.

PER SERVING: Calories: 340; Fat: 13g; Carbohydrates: 31g; Fiber: 8g; Sugar: 12g; Protein: 24g; Sodium: 480mg

TO MAKE THE MEATBALLS

1. In a medium bowl, mix together the beef, bread crumbs, cheese, milk, egg, parsley, salt, and pepper.

2. Form the mixture into 12 meatballs.

TO MAKE THE SAUCE

3. Press the sauté button on the electric pressure cooker, allow it to heat up, then add the oil.

4. Add the onion, carrot, and celery. Sauté for 5 minutes, or until softened.

5. Add the oregano, basil, garlic, salt, and pepper. Sauté for 30 seconds, or until fragrant.

6. Add the tomatoes with their juices and the honey. Mix well. Simmer for 8 to 10 minutes, or until thickened.

7. Nestle the meatballs into the sauce. Press the cancel button to stop cooking.

8. Secure the lid, and cook on high pressure for 5 minutes.

9. After cooking, quick release the pressure. Unlock and remove the lid. Serve immediately.

PORK RAGÙ

This version of pork ragù uses the leaner tenderloin cut. A pork shoulder can also be used for a richer ragù; just be sure to adjust the amounts of the other ingredients accordingly based on the size of the cut of pork. Serve this dish over pasta, vegetable noodles, or whole grains, such as Basic Brown Rice (page 142).

1 pound pork tenderloin

1 teaspoon kosher salt

½ teaspoon freshly ground black pepper

2 tablespoons extra-virgin olive oil, divided

1 onion, diced

5 garlic cloves, minced

½ cup white wine

1 (28-ounce) can low-sodium whole tomatoes

½ cup Vegetable Stock (page 148) or store-bought vegetable stock

1 tablespoon Italian seasoning

½ teaspoon fennel seeds

¼ teaspoon red pepper flakes

SERVES 4
DAIRY-FREE, GLUTEN-FREE

Prep Time: 15 minutes
Pressure Cook: 45 minutes
Pressure Level: High
Release: 15 minutes
Natural, then Quick
Total Time: 1 hour
35 minutes

SAVE FOR LATER: Put leftovers in an airtight container, and refrigerate for up to 5 days, or freeze for up to 3 months.

PER SERVING: Calories: 305; Fat: 11g; Carbohydrates: 19g; Fiber: 4g; Sugar: 12g; Protein: 26g; Sodium: 410mg

1. Season the pork with the salt and pepper.

2. Press the sauté button on the electric pressure cooker, allow it to heat up, then add 1 tablespoon of oil.

3. Add the pork, and cook on 2 sides for about 3 minutes per side, or until browned. Remove the pork, and set aside.

4. Heat the remaining 1 tablespoon of oil.

5. Add the onion, and sauté for 2 minutes, or until softened.

6. Add the garlic, and sauté for 30 seconds, or until fragrant.

7. Add the wine, and deglaze: mix well, and scrape up any brown bits on the bottom of the pot.

8. Add the tomatoes with their juices, stock, Italian seasoning, fennel seeds, and red pepper flakes. Mix well.

9. Return the pork to the pot. Press the cancel button to stop cooking.

10. Secure the lid, and cook on high pressure for 45 minutes.

11. After cooking, let the pressure release naturally for 15 minutes, then quick release the remaining pressure. Unlock and remove the lid.

12. Using 2 forks, shred the pork. Serve.

DECONSTRUCTED LAMB-STUFFED CABBAGE

Stuffed cabbage rolls, also known as malfouf, *are a traditional Lebanese dish. I've deconstructed them to create a variation that works well in the electric pressure cooker. Pair this recipe with some roasted sweet potatoes to round out the meal.*

1 tablespoon extra-virgin olive oil

1 pound ground lamb

1 teaspoon kosher salt

¼ teaspoon freshly ground black pepper

1 onion, diced

4 garlic cloves, minced

1 teaspoon sumac

½ teaspoon ground cinnamon

1 head green cabbage, cored and chopped

¾ cup brown rice

½ cup gluten-free beef stock

Juice of 1 lemon

SERVES 4

DAIRY-FREE, GLUTEN-FREE

Prep Time: 20 minutes

Pressure Cook: 20 minutes

Pressure Level: High

Release: 10 minutes Natural, then Quick

Total Time: 1 hour 10 minutes

SIMPLE SWAP: Any ground meat or poultry will work well in this recipe.

PER SERVING: Calories: 340; Fat: 13g; Carbohydrates: 31g; Fiber: 8g; Sugar: 12g; Protein: 24g; Sodium: 480mg

1. Press the sauté button on the electric pressure cooker, allow it to heat up, then add the oil.

2. Add the lamb. Season with the salt and pepper. Cook for about 5 minutes, or until browned.

3. Add the onion, and sauté for 3 minutes, or until softened.

4. Add the garlic, sumac, and cinnamon. Sauté for 30 seconds, or until fragrant.

5. Add the cabbage, rice, and stock. Press the cancel button to stop cooking.

6. Secure the lid, and cook on high pressure for 20 minutes.

7. After cooking, let the pressure release naturally for 10 minutes, then quick release the remaining pressure. Unlock and remove the lid.

8. Add the lemon juice, mix well, then serve.

CHAPTER EIGHT

DESSERT

POACHED PEARS WITH CARDAMOM

Page 132

BAKED APPLES

Apples hold up well in the electric pressure cooker and provide a nice sweet treat. Granny Smith apples are tart and keep their texture well during cooking. However, some other varieties, such as golden delicious and Fuji, are best eaten raw.

4 Granny Smith apples, cored

2 tablespoons raisins

2 tablespoons chopped walnuts

4 teaspoons honey

1 teaspoon ground cinnamon

Olive oil cooking spray, for coating the steam rack

1. Pour 1 cup of water into the electric pressure cooker.

2. Fill the apples with the raisins, walnuts, honey, and cinnamon.

3. Coat the steam rack with cooking spray, and put it inside the pot, handles extending up. Place the apples on the prepared steam rack.

4. Secure the lid, and cook on high pressure for 10 minutes.

5. After cooking, let the pressure release naturally for 15 minutes, then quick release the remaining pressure. Unlock and remove the lid.

6. Carefully remove the steam rack with the apples, and serve warm.

SERVES 4

DAIRY-FREE, GLUTEN-FREE

Prep Time: 15 minutes

Pressure Cook: 10 minutes

Pressure Level: High

Release: 15 minutes Natural, then Quick

Total Time: 50 minutes

SIMPLE SWAP: Swap out the walnuts and raisins for any nuts and dried fruit you like.

PER SERVING: Calories: 180; Fat: 3g; Carbohydrates: 38g; Fiber: 6g; Sugar: 28g; Protein: 2g; Sodium: 5mg

BERRY COMPOTE WITH YOGURT

This dish is a delicious and nutritious dessert, snack, or breakfast. To bump up the fiber content, add a handful of nuts or seeds. Or add a pop of color and flavor with some chopped mint. Berry compote is a great recipe to batch up and keep on hand in the freezer.

2 pounds mixed berries

2 tablespoons maple syrup

2 tablespoons maple sugar

Grated zest of ½ lemon

Juice of ½ lemon

Grated zest of ½ orange

Juice of ½ orange

2 cups Plain Yogurt (page 145) or store-bought plain yogurt

SERVES 4

GLUTEN-FREE

Prep Time: 15 minutes

Pressure Cook: 2 minutes

Pressure Level: High

Release: 15 minutes Natural, then Quick

Total Time: 40 to 45 minutes

SAVE FOR LATER: The berry compote can be stored in an airtight container for up to 1 week in the refrigerator or up to 6 months in the freezer.

PER SERVING: Calories: 220; Fat: 3g; Carbohydrates: 43g; Fiber: 10g; Sugar: 30g; Protein: 8g; Sodium: 240mg

1. In the electric pressure cooker, combine the berries, maple syrup, maple sugar, lemon zest, lemon juice, orange zest, and orange juice. Mix well.

2. Secure the lid, and cook on high pressure for 2 minutes.

3. After cooking, let the pressure release naturally for 15 minutes, then quick release the remaining pressure. Unlock and remove the lid, then mix well.

4. If desired, press the sauté button, and simmer the mixture to thicken. Press the cancel button to stop cooking.

5. Serve the compote with the yogurt.

POACHED PEARS WITH CARDAMOM

Poached pears are one of my favorite fruit-based desserts. My version uses white wine and cardamom, adding spicy, herbal, fragrant notes to the dish. If you do not have cardamom, try a 1-inch knob of peeled ginger and a cinnamon stick instead. Red wine may also be used in place of the white wine if preferred.

4 firm pears, peeled

2 cups water

2 cups dry white wine

½ cup granulated sugar

2 tablespoons freshly squeezed lemon juice

10 cardamom pods, lightly crushed, or 1 teaspoon ground cardamom

Pinch saffron threads

⅛ teaspoon kosher salt

½ cup pistachios, toasted and chopped

SERVES 4

DAIRY-FREE, GLUTEN-FREE

Prep Time: 10 minutes

Pressure Cook: 8 minutes

Pressure Level: High

Release: Quick

Total Time: 45 minutes

SIMPLE SWAP: If you don't have pistachios, use any nuts or seeds you like. You can also top the pears with a dollop of yogurt, crème fraîche, or whipped cream in addition to or in place of the nuts.

PER SERVING: Calories: 260; Fat: 7g; Carbohydrates: 43g; Fiber: 6g; Sugar: 35g; Protein: 4g; Sodium: 38mg

1. Using a melon baller or spoon, scoop out the seeds and core from the bottom of each pear.

2. In the electric pressure cooker, combine the water, wine, sugar, lemon juice, cardamom, saffron, and salt. Mix well. Press the sauté button, and bring to a simmer.

3. Add the pears, and press the cancel button to stop cooking.

4. Secure the lid, and cook on high pressure for 8 minutes.

5. After cooking, quick release the pressure. Unlock and remove the lid.

6. Transfer the pears to serving dishes.

7. Press the sauté button, and bring the liquid to a boil. Reduce by about half. Press the cancel button to stop cooking.

8. While the liquid boils, in a small skillet, toast the pistachios over medium heat for about 5 minutes, or until golden brown. Remove from the heat.

9. Ladle the sauce over each pear, and garnish with the pistachios.

CHOCOLATE POT DE CRÈME

These sweet treats are sure to be a crowd-pleaser. Serve them with berries and a dollop of crème fraîche or Plain Yogurt (page 145) and some fresh mint. I like using maple sugar because it adds a nice flavor to the dish, but feel free to swap it out for brown sugar or coconut sugar.

1½ cups heavy cream, divided

2 ounces dark chocolate (70 percent), chopped

Pinch cayenne pepper

4 large egg yolks

3 tablespoons maple sugar

1 teaspoon vanilla extract

¼ teaspoon kosher salt

SERVES 4

GLUTEN-FREE

Prep Time: 15 minutes

Pressure Cook: 8 minutes

Pressure Level: High

Release: 20 minutes Natural, then Quick

Total Time: 1 hour 55 minutes

SIMPLE SWAP: If you prefer milk chocolate or white chocolate, feel free to swap out the dark chocolate.

PER SERVING: Calories: 475; Fat: 44g; Carbohydrates: 16g; Fiber: 2g; Sugar: 12g; Protein: 6g; Sodium: 115mg

1. In a small saucepan, combine ¼ cup of heavy cream and the chocolate. Melt together over low heat, whisking occasionally. Remove from the heat.

2. Whisk in the remaining 1¼ cups of heavy cream and the cayenne.

3. In a medium bowl, whisk together the egg yolks, maple sugar, vanilla, and salt.

4. Whisking continuously, slowly add some of the chocolate-cream mixture until everything is combined. Pour into 4 ramekins, and cover each tightly with aluminum foil.

5. Pour 1½ cups of water into the electric pressure cooker. Put a steam rack inside the pot, handles extending up. Place the ramekins on the steam rack.

6. Secure the lid, and cook on high pressure for 8 minutes.

7. After cooking, let the pressure release naturally for 20 minutes, then quick release the remaining pressure. Unlock and remove the lid.

8. Carefully remove the ramekins, remove the foil, and cool before serving.

NUT AND FIG "PUDDING" WITH YOGURT CREAM

Fig trees are native to the Mediterranean region and are also the world's first cultivated tree. Figs vary in color and texture depending on the variety, ranging from light green to purple or yellow skin and pink to amber or red flesh. Some of the most popular fig types are black mission, Calimyrna, brown turkey, and Adriatic.

FOR THE PUDDING

1 pound figs, stemmed and chopped

1 cup water

½ cup chopped walnuts

½ cup chopped pistachios

½ cup chopped pecans

¼ cup ground espresso (optional)

3 tablespoons unsalted butter, melted

½ teaspoon ground cardamom

¼ teaspoon ground ginger

¼ teaspoon ground cinnamon

¼ teaspoon kosher salt

FOR THE YOGURT CREAM

½ cup heavy cream

¼ cup Plain Yogurt (page 145) or store-bought plain yogurt

1 teaspoon confectioner's sugar

TO MAKE THE PUDDING

1. In the electric pressure cooker, combine the figs and water. Secure the lid, and cook on high pressure for 5 minutes.

2. After cooking, quick release the pressure. Unlock and remove the lid.

SERVES 6

GLUTEN-FREE

Prep Time: 15 minutes

Pressure Cook: 5 minutes

Pressure Level: High

Release: Quick

Total Time: 40 to 45 minutes

SIMPLE SWAP: Feel free to swap out any of the nuts and use whatever nuts and seeds you like.

PER SERVING: Calories: 370; Fat: 31g; Carbohydrates: 22g; Fiber: 5g; Sugar: 15g; Protein: 6g; Sodium: 65mg

3. Mash together the figs and water.

4. Add the walnuts, pistachios, pecans, espresso (if using), butter, cardamom, ginger, cinnamon, and salt. Press the sauté button, and simmer, stirring often, for 10 minutes, or until thickened. Press the cancel button to stop cooking.

TO MAKE THE YOGURT CREAM

5. In a medium bowl, combine the heavy cream, yogurt, and sugar. Whisk for about 2 minutes, or until soft peaks form.

6. Divide the pudding among bowls. Top with the yogurt cream.

CUSTARD WITH ROASTED FRUIT

Roasted fruit is amazingly delicious on its own, but it pairs beautifully with this custard. You can make the custard the day before and serve it chilled with warm roasted fruit. Basil also goes nicely with this dessert in place of the mint.

FOR THE CUSTARD

1¾ cups whole milk

4 large eggs

3 tablespoons granulated sugar

1 teaspoon vanilla extract

¼ teaspoon kosher salt

FOR THE ROASTED FRUIT

1 tablespoon maple syrup

1 teaspoon extra-virgin olive oil

¼ teaspoon kosher salt

½ cup strawberries, stemmed

½ cup raspberries

¼ cup chopped fresh mint leaves

SERVES 4

GLUTEN-FREE

Prep Time: 15 minutes

Pressure Cook: 6 minutes

Pressure Level: High

Release: 20 minutes Natural, then Quick

Total Time: 1 hour 30 minutes

SIMPLE SWAP: For a delicious twist, swap out the vanilla extract for almond extract.

PER SERVING: Calories: 160; Fat: 5g; Carbohydrates: 22g; Fiber: 2g; Sugar: 20g; Protein: 7g; Sodium: 250mg

TO MAKE THE CUSTARD

1. In a medium bowl, whisk together the milk, eggs, sugar, vanilla, and salt. Pour into 4 ramekins, and cover tightly with aluminum foil.

2. Pour 1½ cups of water into the electric pressure cooker. Put a steam rack inside the pot, handles extending up. Place the ramekins on the steam rack.

3. Secure the lid, and cook on high pressure for 6 minutes.

4. After cooking, let the pressure release naturally for 20 minutes, then quick release the remaining pressure. Unlock and remove the lid.

5. Carefully remove the ramekins, remove the foil, and let cool.

TO MAKE THE ROASTED FRUIT

6. While the custard is cooking, preheat the oven to 250°F. Line a baking sheet with parchment paper or foil.

7. In a large bowl, whisk together the maple syrup, oil, and salt.

8. Add the berries, and carefully toss together.

9. Spread the berries out in a single layer on the prepared baking sheet.

10. Transfer the baking sheet to the oven, and roast for 1 hour 30 minutes, or until the fruit is reduced and soft. Remove from the oven.

11. Serve the custard with the roasted fruit, and garnish with the mint.

RICE PUDDING

Rice pudding can be found throughout the Mediterranean, taking on slightly different flavors and variations depending on the region. Some areas use nutmeg or cardamom in addition to the cinnamon, and others use orange blossom water or rose water. Regardless of where you are, the basics of rice pudding remain the same. Feel free to experiment and see what add-ins you like!

1 tablespoon unsalted butter

⅔ cup Arborio rice

1 (12-ounce) can evaporated reduced fat milk

½ cup water

⅓ cup maple sugar

1 cinnamon stick

1 tablespoon granulated sugar

1 teaspoon vanilla extract

¼ teaspoon kosher salt

¼ cup heavy cream

1 large egg

1 large egg yolk

SERVES 4

GLUTEN-FREE

Prep Time: 15 minutes

Pressure Cook: 10 minutes

Pressure Level: High

Release: 15 minutes Natural, then Quick

Total Time: 1 hour 5 minutes

TROUBLESHOOTING TIP: Add the hot rice mixture carefully to the egg mixture, being sure to temper properly and not scramble the egg. This can be done by adding a small amount at a time and mixing well before adding more.

PER SERVING: Calories: 355; Fat: 13g; Carbohydrates: 48g; Fiber: 1g; Sugar: 19g; Protein: 12g; Sodium: 200mg

1. Press the sauté button on the electric pressure cooker, allow it to heat up, then add the butter.

2. Once the butter has melted, add the rice, and sauté for 1 minute.

3. Add the evaporated milk, water, maple sugar, cinnamon, sugar, vanilla, and salt. Mix well. Press the cancel button to stop cooking.

4. Secure the lid, and cook on high pressure for 10 minutes.

5. After cooking, let the pressure release naturally for 15 minutes, then quick release the remaining pressure. Unlock and remove the lid, then mix well. Remove the cinnamon stick.

6. In a small bowl, whisk together the heavy cream, egg, and egg yolk.

7. Add ½ cup of the rice mixture to the egg mixture, and mix vigorously.

8. Add the egg and rice mixture to the rest of the rice, and mix together well. Let sit for 5 to 10 minutes.

9. Serve warm, or transfer to airtight containers and chill in the refrigerator before serving.

CHAPTER NINE

SAUCES AND STAPLES

BASIL-WALNUT PESTO Page 150

BASIC BROWN RICE

Brown rice is a wonderfully versatile grain able to complement practically any food. There are many different varieties of rice, but brown rice is one of the most nutritious. It is chock-full of B vitamins, manganese, selenium, iron, dietary fiber, and protein in addition to many other nutrients.

1 tablespoon extra-virgin olive oil

1½ cups long-grain brown rice, rinsed

1 teaspoon kosher salt

6 cups water

MAKES 3 CUPS
DAIRY-FREE, GLUTEN-FREE

Prep Time: 5 minutes

Pressure Cook: 15 minutes

Pressure Level: Low

Release: 20 minutes Natural, then Quick

Total Time: 45 to 50 minutes

1. Press the sauté button on the electric pressure cooker, allow it to heat up, then add the oil.

2. Add the rice and salt. Sauté for 30 seconds.

3. Add the water, and mix well. Press the cancel button to stop cooking.

4. Secure the lid, and cook on low pressure for 15 minutes.

5. After cooking, let the pressure release naturally for 20 minutes, then quick release the remaining pressure. Unlock and remove the lid.

6. Mix well, and taste for doneness. If there is liquid remaining in the pot, drain it through a fine-mesh strainer.

SAVE FOR LATER: To save rice, first spread it on a rimmed baking sheet to cool to room temperature quickly. Store it in airtight containers or resealable freezer bags, label with the name and date, and put in the refrigerator for up to 1 week or in the freezer for up to 3 months.

PER SERVING (½ CUP): Calories: 190; Fat: 4g; Carbohydrates: 37g; Fiber: 3g; Sugar: 0g; Protein: 3g; Sodium: 200mg

BASIC BEANS

Beans are a staple throughout the Mediterranean region and are an excellent source of plant-based protein. Most dried beans, including chickpeas, cannellini beans, and kidney beans, should take 30 minutes to cook; however, if you open the lid and find your beans still a bit too hard for your liking, simply turn on the sauté function and simmer for 5 to 10 minutes.

6 cups water

1 pound dried beans of choice, picked through and rinsed

½ teaspoon kosher salt

1. In the electric pressure cooker, combine the water, beans, and salt. Secure the lid, and cook on high pressure for 30 minutes.

2. After cooking, let the pressure release naturally for 30 minutes, then quick release the remaining pressure. Unlock and remove the lid, then mix well.

MAKES 6 CUPS

DAIRY-FREE, GLUTEN-FREE

Prep Time: 5 minutes

Pressure Cook: 30 minutes

Pressure Level: High

Release: 30 minutes Natural, then Quick

Total Time: 1 hour 15 minutes

SAVE FOR LATER: Store beans in airtight containers, with or without liquid, for up to 1 week in the refrigerator or up to 6 months in the freezer.

PER SERVING (½ CUP): Calories: 125; Fat: 0g; Carbohydrates: 23g; Fiber: 9g; Sugar: 1g; Protein: 9g; Sodium: 60mg

HARD- AND SOFT-BOILED EGGS

Eggs are an excellent source of protein, clocking in at 6 grams per large egg. They also have many essential vitamins and minerals, including vitamin B$_{12}$, choline, selenium, and biotin. Making a dozen hard-boiled eggs in the electric pressure cooker is a breeze. Keep them in the refrigerator to add to meals and snacks all week.

6 large eggs

1. Fill a large bowl with ice water.

2. Pour 1 cup of water into the electric pressure cooker. Put a steam rack in the pot, and place the eggs carefully on top. Secure the lid, and cook on high pressure for 3 minutes (soft-boiled), 4 to 5 minutes (medium-boiled), or 6 to 7 minutes (hard-boiled).

3. After cooking, quick release the pressure. Unlock and remove the lid.

4. Transfer the eggs immediately to the ice water bath for 1 to 2 minutes.

SERVES 6

DAIRY-FREE, GLUTEN-FREE

Prep Time: 5 minutes

Pressure Cook: 3 to 7 minutes

Pressure Level: High

Release: Quick

Total Time: 15 to 25 minutes

SAVE FOR LATER: If not eating right away, leave in shell, and refrigerate for up to 5 days.

PER SERVING (1 EGG):
Calories: 70; Fat: 5g; Carbohydrates: 0g; Fiber: 0g; Sugar: 0g; Protein: 6g; Sodium: 70mg

PLAIN YOGURT

Yogurt is a staple in the Mediterranean diet and, like other dairy products, is a very good source of protein, calcium, phosphorous, vitamin B_{12}, and many other nutrients. Yogurt is a fermented dairy product, meaning it is made by adding bacterial cultures to milk that convert the lactose into lactic acid. This process creates yogurt's tart and sour flavor and unique texture. As you'll see from the recipe, the process takes some time but is very easy to do—and well worth the wait!

5 cups reduced fat or whole milk

2 tablespoons plain yogurt (with live cultures)

1. Pour the milk into the electric pressure cooker. Secure the lid, press the yogurt button, and adjust the pressure to boil. This part takes about 30 minutes.

2. Once done, fill a large bowl with ice water. Remove the entire pot, and place it in the ice water bath for 15 minutes, or until the milk chills to 100°F to 115°F.

3. Add the yogurt to the milk, and whisk.

4. Remove the pot from the ice bath, dry it off, and place back in the electric pressure cooker.

5. Press the yogurt button, and set the timer to 8 hours.

6. After cooking, transfer the yogurt to airtight containers, and refrigerate for 8 to 10 hours before eating.

MAKES 5 CUPS

GLUTEN-FREE

Prep Time: 10 minutes

Pressure Cook: 8 hours 30 minutes

Pressure Level: Yogurt

Total Time: 9 hours, plus at least 8 hours to chill

SAVE FOR LATER: Yogurt can be stored in airtight containers in the refrigerator for up to 10 days or in the freezer for up to 1 month.

PER SERVING (½ CUP):
Calories: 65; Fat: 2g;
Carbohydrates: 6g; Fiber: 0g;
Sugar: 6g; Protein: 4g;
Sodium: 60mg

HUMMUS

Hummus is a staple throughout the Mediterranean region. There are many different variations, such as adding spices like Za'atar and sumac or incorporating ingredients like roasted red peppers. Drizzle some nice olive oil on top, and serve with pita bread and crudités.

2 cups Basic Chickpeas (page 143) or canned chickpeas

⅓ cup tahini

Juice of 1 lemon

1 garlic clove, smashed and peeled

1 teaspoon kosher salt

½ teaspoon ground cumin

¼ teaspoon freshly ground black pepper

3 tablespoons extra-virgin olive oil

MAKES ABOUT 2 CUPS

DAIRY-FREE, GLUTEN-FREE

Prep Time: 15 minutes

Total Time: 15 minutes

SIMPLE SWAP: Traditional hummus uses chickpeas, but other beans also taste great and work well in this recipe.

PER SERVING (¼ CUP):
Calories: 170; Fat: 11g;
Carbohydrates: 14g;
Fiber: 4g; Sugar: 2g;
Protein: 5g; Sodium: 150mg

1. In a food processor, combine the chickpeas, tahini, lemon juice, garlic, salt, cumin, and pepper. Pulse 8 to 10 times.

2. Continue to process while adding the oil until the desired consistency is reached.

TZATZIKI

I love the refreshing mix of cucumbers, yogurt, and herbs. And the zingy lemon makes the whole dish pop! Here's a tip: grate the cucumber using the large holes of a box grater for a chunkier version or the small holes for a smoother version. Pair this with pita bread, vegetables, or roasted meat or poultry.

2 Persian cucumbers, grated

1 cup Plain Yogurt (page 145) or store-bought plain yogurt

2 tablespoons chopped fresh dill

2 tablespoons chopped fresh mint leaves

Juice of ½ lemon

1 tablespoon extra-virgin olive oil

1 garlic clove, grated

¾ teaspoon kosher salt

MAKES 1½ CUPS
GLUTEN-FREE

Prep Time: 15 minutes
Total Time: 15 minutes

SAVE FOR LATER: Tzatziki should stay fresh in the refrigerator for up to 5 days. Just give it a good stir before serving.

PER SERVING (¼ CUP): Calories: 55; Fat: 3g; Carbohydrates: 5g; Fiber: 0g; Sugar: 4g; Protein: 2g; Sodium: 175mg

In a medium bowl, combine the cucumbers, yogurt, dill, mint, lemon juice, oil, garlic, and salt. Mix together well.

VEGETABLE STOCK

Homemade vegetable stock is amazingly flavorful and easy to make and have on hand. During the week, simply save leftover vegetable scraps, put them in a resealable bag, and freeze. Once you have enough vegetables saved up, you can add them to this recipe.

2 onions, quartered

2 carrots, quartered

2 celery stalks, cut into 2-inch pieces

1 bunch parsley

6 thyme sprigs

5 garlic cloves, smashed and peeled

1½ teaspoons kosher salt

1 teaspoon black peppercorns

3 bay leaves

10 cups water

MAKES 10 CUPS

DAIRY-FREE, GLUTEN-FREE

Prep Time: 15 minutes

Pressure Cook: 1 hour

Pressure Level: High

Release: 30 minutes Natural, then Quick

Total Time: 2 hours 25 minutes

1. In the electric pressure cooker, combine the onions, carrots, celery, parsley, thyme, garlic, salt, peppercorns, and bay leaves.

2. Add the water, making sure not to go past the "max fill" line. Secure the lid, and cook on high pressure for 1 hour.

3. After cooking, let the pressure release naturally for 30 minutes, then quick release the remaining pressure. Unlock and remove the lid, then mix well.

4. Strain the stock through a fine-mesh strainer or colander into a large bowl. Discard the solids, and cool the stock for 30 minutes.

SAVE FOR LATER: Portion out vegetable stock into airtight containers, and store in the refrigerator for up to 1 week or in the freezer for up to 6 months. If freezing, you can portion out stock into resealable freezer bags and place several in a stack flat on a baking sheet. Once frozen, remove the baking sheet, and keep the frozen stock stacked in the freezer.

PER SERVING (½ CUP): Calories: 0; Fat: 0g; Carbohydrates: 0g; Fiber: 0g; Sugar: 0g; Protein: 0g; Sodium: 90mg

CHICKEN STOCK

Homemade chicken stock is always useful in the kitchen, so I like to have several quart containers in the freezer at all times. Make the Whole Chicken (page 112), then cut off all the meat and use the carcass (wings, neck, backs, leftover carcass) to make this delicious, simple chicken stock.

2 to 2½ pounds chicken bones

1 onion, quartered

2 carrots, quartered

2 celery stalks, cut into 2-inch pieces

3 garlic cloves, smashed and peeled

1½ teaspoons kosher salt

1 teaspoon black peppercorns

3 bay leaves

10 cups water

MAKES 10 CUPS

DAIRY-FREE, GLUTEN-FREE

Prep Time: 15 minutes

Pressure Cook: 1 hour

Pressure Level: High

Release: 30 minutes Natural, then Quick

Total Time: 2 hours 25 minutes

1. In the electric pressure cooker, combine the chicken bones, onion, carrots, celery, garlic, salt, peppercorns, and bay leaves.

2. Add the water, making sure not to go past the "max fill" line. Secure the lid, and cook on high pressure for 1 hour.

3. After cooking, let the pressure release naturally for 30 minutes, then quick release the remaining pressure. Unlock and remove the lid, then mix well.

4. Strain the stock through a fine-mesh strainer or colander into a large bowl. Discard the solids, and cool the stock for 30 minutes.

SAVE FOR LATER: Portion out chicken stock into airtight containers, and store in the refrigerator for up to 1 week or in the freezer for up to 3 months. If freezing, you can portion out stock into resealable freezer bags and place several in a stack flat on a baking sheet. Once frozen, remove the baking sheet, and keep the frozen stock stacked in the freezer.

PER SERVING (½ CUP):
Calories: 0; Fat: 0g; Carbohydrates: 0g; Fiber: 0g; Sugar: 0g; Protein: 0g; Sodium: 90mg

BASIL-WALNUT PESTO

Pesto is one of my go-to secrets when I need to add a pop of flavor to a dish. This version is slightly different than a classic version, with walnuts taking the place of pine nuts. You can easily adjust the recipe to include whatever herbs and nuts you have on hand. For a spicy kick, add a pinch of red pepper flakes! This versatile pesto tastes great paired with pasta, fish, meat, poultry, and roasted vegetables.

2 cups loosely packed fresh basil leaves

⅓ cup chopped walnuts

⅓ cup grated Parmesan cheese

1 garlic clove, peeled

½ teaspoon kosher salt

¼ teaspoon freshly ground black pepper

⅓ cup extra-virgin olive oil

MAKES 1 CUP

GLUTEN-FREE

Prep Time: 10 minutes

Total Time: 10 minutes

1. In a food processor, combine the basil, walnuts, cheese, garlic, salt, and pepper. Pulse 8 to 10 times.

2. Continue to process while adding the oil until the desired consistency is reached.

SAVE FOR LATER: Freeze any leftover pesto in ice cube trays. Simply pop out the pesto cubes once they're frozen, and store in a resealable freezer bag. You'll be able to grab a perfectly portioned pesto cube any time and add it to your favorite meals!

PER SERVING (2 TABLESPOONS):
Calories: 175; Fat: 18g; Carbohydrates: 2g; Fiber: 1g; Sugar: 0g; Protein: 4g; Sodium: 175mg

TAHINI DRESSING

This delightful tahini dressing goes well as a salad dressing; can be drizzled over roasted vegetables, meat, or poultry; and can even be used as a dipping sauce. It will stay fresh in the refrigerator for up to 2 weeks. Simply remove from the refrigerator a few minutes before serving to allow it to come to room temperature, then shake or whisk well.

1 cup extra-virgin olive oil

½ cup water

⅓ cup tahini

¼ cup tamari

¼ cup freshly squeezed lemon juice

2 tablespoons sesame oil

1½ teaspoons dry mustard

¾ teaspoon kosher salt

⅛ teaspoon cayenne pepper

In a medium bowl, whisk together the olive oil, water, tahini, tamari, lemon juice, sesame oil, mustard, salt, and cayenne. (You can also use an immersion blender.)

MAKES 2 CUPS
DAIRY-FREE, GLUTEN-FREE

Prep Time: 10 minutes
Total Time: 10 minutes

SIMPLE SWAP: Tamari is gluten-free soy sauce, but if you are not following a gluten-free diet, feel free to use low-sodium soy sauce in its place.

PER SERVING (2 TABLESPOONS):
Calories: 165; Fat: 18g; Carbohydrates: 2g; Fiber: 1g; Sugar: 0g; Protein: 1g; Sodium: 310mg

PRESSURE COOKING CHARTS

These charts are intended to be used as helpful cooking aids for those looking to do more in the kitchen with their electric pressure cooker and have been included as a resourceful guide to cooking the basics, not just the recipes in this book.

Beans and Legumes

While the recipes in this book call for unsoaked beans, for those interested in cooking soaked beans in their electric pressure cooker, the cooking times below are for beans that have been soaked for 8 to 24 hours in salted water, unless otherwise noted.

	MINUTES UNDER PRESSURE	PRESSURE	RELEASE
BLACK BEANS	8	High	Natural for 15 to 20 minutes, then quick
BLACK-EYED PEAS	5	High	Natural for 15 to 20 minutes, then quick
CANNELLINI BEANS	5	High	Natural for 15 to 20 minutes, then quick
CHICKPEAS (GARBANZO BEANS)	4	High	Natural for 15 to 20 minutes, then quick
KIDNEY BEANS	5	High	Natural for 15 to 20 minutes, then quick
BROWN LENTILS (UNSOAKED)	20	High	Natural for 10 minutes, then quick
RED LENTILS (UNSOAKED)	10	High	Natural for 5 minutes, then quick
PINTO BEANS	8	High	Natural for 15 to 20 minutes, then quick
SPLIT PEAS (UNSOAKED)	8	High	Natural for 15 to 20 minutes, then quick
LIMA BEANS	4	High	Natural for 15 to 20 minutes, then quick
SOYBEANS, FRESH (EDAMAME), UNSOAKED	1	High	Quick
SOYBEANS, DRIED	12	High	Natural for 15 to 20 minutes, then quick

Grains

To prevent foaming, rinse grains thoroughly before cooking.

	LIQUID PER 1 CUP OF GRAIN	MINUTES UNDER PRESSURE	PRESSURE	RELEASE
ARBORIO RICE (FOR RISOTTO)	3 to 4 cups	6 to 8	High	Natural for 15 minutes, then quick
BARLEY, PEARLED	2½ cups	20	High	Natural for 10 minutes, then quick
BROWN RICE, MEDIUM-GRAIN	1 cup	15	Low	Natural for 15 to 20 minutes, then quick
BROWN RICE, LONG-GRAIN	1 cup	15	Low	Natural for 20 minutes, then quick
BUCKWHEAT	1¾ cups	2 to 4	High	Natural for 15 to 20 minutes, then quick
FARRO, WHOLE-GRAIN	3 cups	22 to 24	High	Natural for 15 to 20 minutes, then quick
FARRO, PEARLED	2 cups	6 to 8	High	Natural for 15 to 20 minutes, then quick
OATS, ROLLED	3 cups	3 to 4	High	Quick
OATS, STEEL-CUT	3 cups	10	High	Natural for 10 minutes, then quick
QUINOA	1½ cups	1	High	Natural for 15 minutes, then Quick
WHEAT BERRIES	2 cups	30	High	Natural for 10 minutes, then quick
WHITE RICE, LONG-GRAIN	1 cup	3	High	Natural for 15 to 20 minutes, then quick
WILD RICE	1¼ cups	22 to 24	High	Natural for 15 to 20 minutes, then quick

Meat

Except as noted, these times are for braised meats: that is, meats that are seared before pressure cooking and partially submerged in liquid.

	MINUTES UNDER PRESSURE	PRESSURE	RELEASE
BEEF, BONE-IN SHORT RIBS	40	High	Natural for 30 to 40 minutes
BEEF, FLAT IRON STEAK, CUT INTO ½-INCH STRIPS	6	Low	Quick
BEEF, SHOULDER (CHUCK) ROAST (2 POUNDS)	35 to 45	High	Natural for 30 to 40 minutes
BEEF, SHOULDER (CHUCK), 2-INCH CHUNKS	20	High	Natural for 10 minutes
BEEF, SIRLOIN STEAK, CUT INTO ½-INCH STRIPS	3	Low	Quick
LAMB, SHANKS	45	High	Natural for 30 to 40 minutes
LAMB, SHOULDER, 2-INCH CHUNKS	35	High	Natural for 30 to 40 minutes
PORK, BACK RIBS (STEAMED)	25	High	Quick
PORK, SHOULDER ROAST (2 POUNDS)	25	High	Natural for 30 to 40 minutes
PORK, SHOULDER, 2-INCH CHUNKS	20	High	Quick
PORK, SPARE RIBS (STEAMED)	20	High	Quick
PORK, TENDERLOIN	4	Low	Quick
SMOKED PORK SAUSAGE, ½-INCH SLICES	5 to 10	High	Quick

Poultry

Except as noted, these times are for braised poultry: that is, partially submerged in liquid.

	MINUTES UNDER PRESSURE	PRESSURE	RELEASE
CHICKEN BREAST, BONE-IN	15	High	Quick
CHICKEN BREAST, BONELESS	5 (steamed)	Low	Natural for 8 minutes
CHICKEN THIGH, BONE-IN	15 to 25	High	Natural for 20 minutes
CHICKEN THIGH, BONELESS	15 to 25	High	Natural for 20 minutes
CHICKEN, WHOLE	30	High	Natural for 15 minutes
DUCK QUARTERS, BONE-IN	35	High	Quick
TURKEY BREAST, TENDERLOIN, 12 OUNCES	5 (steamed)	Low	Natural for 8 minutes
TURKEY THIGH, BONE-IN	30	High	Natural for 20 minutes

Fish and Seafood

All times are for steamed fish and shellfish.

	MINUTES UNDER PRESSURE	PRESSURE	RELEASE
CLAMS	4	High	Natural for 15 minutes, then quick
HALIBUT (1-INCH THICK)	3	High	Quick
MUSSELS	2	High	Quick
SALMON (1-INCH THICK)	3	Low	Quick
SHRIMP, LARGE (FROZEN)	1	Low	Quick
TILAPIA OR COD	3	Low	Quick

Vegetables

The cooking method for all the following vegetables is steaming; if the vegetables are cooked in liquid, the times may vary. Green vegetables will be tender-crisp; root vegetables will be soft.

	PREP	MINUTES UNDER PRESSURE	PRESSURE	RELEASE
ACORN SQUASH	Halved	9	High	Quick
ARTICHOKES, LARGE	Whole	8	High	Quick
BEETS	Whole	20	High	Quick
BROCCOLI	Cut into florets	0 to 1	Low	Quick
BRUSSELS SPROUTS	Halved	2	High	Quick
BUTTERNUT SQUASH	Peeled, cut into ½-inch chunks	8	High	Quick
CABBAGE	Sliced	3 to 4	High	Quick
CARROTS	½- to 1-inch slices	2	High	Quick
CAULIFLOWER	Whole	6	High	Quick
CAULIFLOWER	Cut into florets	0 to 1	Low	Quick
GREEN BEANS	Cut in half or thirds	0 to 3	Low	Quick
POTATOES, LARGE RUSSET	Quartered; for mashing	8	High	Natural for 8 minutes, then quick
POTATOES, RED	Whole if less than 1½ inch across, halved if larger	4	High	Quick
SPAGHETTI SQUASH	Halved lengthwise	7	High	Quick
SWEET POTATOES	Halved lengthwise	12	High	Quick

MEASUREMENT CONVERSIONS

VOLUME EQUIVALENTS	U.S. STANDARD	U.S. STANDARD (ounces)	METRIC (approximate)
LIQUID	2 tablespoons	1 fl. oz.	30 mL
	¼ cup	2 fl. oz.	60 mL
	½ cup	4 fl. oz.	120 mL
	1 cup	8 fl. oz.	240 mL
	1½ cups	12 fl. oz.	355 mL
	2 cups or 1 pint	16 fl. oz.	475 mL
	4 cups or 1 quart	32 fl. oz.	1 L
	1 gallon	128 fl. oz.	4 L
DRY	⅛ teaspoon	—	0.5 mL
	¼ teaspoon	—	1 mL
	½ teaspoon	—	2 mL
	¾ teaspoon	—	4 mL
	1 teaspoon	—	5 mL
	1 tablespoon	—	15 mL
	¼ cup	—	59 mL
	⅓ cup	—	79 mL
	½ cup	—	118 mL
	⅔ cup	—	156 mL
	¾ cup	—	177 mL
	1 cup	—	235 mL
	2 cups or 1 pint	—	475 mL
	3 cups	—	700 mL
	4 cups or 1 quart	—	1 L
	½ gallon	—	2 L
	1 gallon	—	4 L

Oven Temperatures

FAHRENHEIT	CELSIUS (approximate)
250°F	120°C
300°F	150°C
325°F	165°C
350°F	180°C
375°F	190°C
400°F	200°C
425°F	220°C
450°F	230°C

Weight Equivalents

U.S. STANDARD	METRIC (approximate)
½ ounce	15 g
1 ounce	30 g
2 ounces	60 g
4 ounces	115 g
8 ounces	225 g
12 ounces	340 g
16 ounces or 1 pound	455 g

REFERENCE

Yu, Zhi, Vasanti S. Malik, NaNa Keum, Frank B. Hu, Edward L. Giovannucci, Meir J. Stampfer, Walter C. Willett, et al. "Associations Between Nut Consumption and Inflammatory Biomarkers." *The American Journal of Clinical Nutrition* 104, no. 3 (September 2016): 722–28. doi.org/10.3945/ajcn.116.134205.

INDEX

ABOUT THE AUTHOR

Chef Abbie Gellman, MS, RD, CDN, is a spokesperson, recipe and product developer, and educator. She creates, produces, and hosts cooking and nutrition videos and works with a wide variety of food companies, brands, commodity boards, food service operators, health professionals, and private clients. She also contributes to many publications. Her first cookbook, *The Mediterranean DASH Diet Cookbook*, was published November 2019. She is regularly featured in the media, where she shares culinary nutrition expertise and delicious, nutritious recipes. Abbie lives in New York City with her daughter, Olivia, and many shelves of cookbooks. Learn more about her at ChefAbbieGellman.com, and connect with her via @ChefAbbieGellman on Instagram, Chef Abbie Gellman on YouTube and Facebook, and ChefAbbieGellman on Pinterest.

CPSIA information can be obtained
at www.ICGtesting.com
Printed in the USA
JSHW050336171220
10281JS00001B/1